The STARK REALITY of STRETCHING

AN INFORMED
APPROACH FOR ALL
ACTIVITIES AND
EVERY SPORT

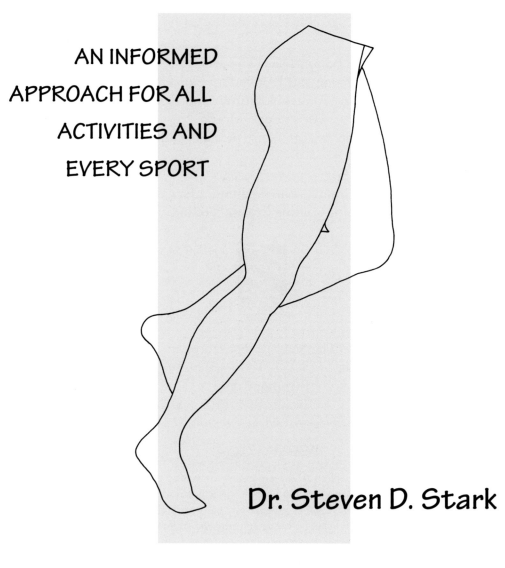

Dr. Steven D. Stark

Canadian Cataloguing in Publication Data
Stark, Steven D. (Steven Daryl), 1948–
The Stark reality of stretching: an informed
approach for all activities and every sport.
4th ed., rev.
Includes bibliographical references.
ISBN 0-9683607-1-8
1. Stretching exercises. I. Title.
GV505.S72 1999   613.7'1   C99-901329-7

Editor: Diana C. Douglas
Book Design and Production: Fiona Raven
Cover Design: Andrew Johnstone and Fiona Raven
Artist: Susie Morris
Title, Subtitle, Cover Design Concepts, and Editing: Sylvia Stark

First printing October 1997
Fourth printing, revised edition, October 1999
Fifth printing September 2006

The Stark Reality Corp.
Suite 1115-11871 Horseshoe Way
Richmond, BC
Canada V7A 5H5
Phone 604-538-5074 or Fax 604-538-5063

Printed in Canada

Consult your physician before beginning any exercise or stretching program if you have any health problems or injuries. Before engaging in these stretches, read the entire book to become familiar with all the information. If you experience any pain while doing these stretches do not continue to stretch. See your physician before attempting the stretches again.

This publication is designed to provide accurate and authoritative information in regard to the subject matter covered. It is sold with the understanding that the author, publisher, editors and distributors are not engaged in rendering medical or professional service.

DEDICATION

This book is dedicated to my partner
in life, my biggest supporter, my
harshest critic, my balance, my love —

my wife Sylvia

ACKNOWLEDGMENTS

My thanks to Diana Douglas, organizer and editor supreme, for her guidance in making this project a reality. The book design artist, Fiona Raven, has contributed greatly in making this book user friendly and effective. The illustrations give life to a difficult subject, thanks to our artist, Susie Morris. The continuing evolution of cover design and text is the computer magic of Andrew Johnstone.

Thank you all.

PREFACE

If you watch my TV show "Everyday Workout" you have been using some of Dr. Steven Stark's techniques already! As the host of one of North America's top exercise programs, my audience expects me to give them the correct information about stretching.

I use many of the techniques Dr. Stark presents in *The Stark Reality of Stretching* consistently with my viewers. There are many misconceptions about how muscles work and how to keep our body tuned and lessen potential injuries. This book not only describes how your lower body works but also why stretching the wrong way can actually contribute to more exercise problems.

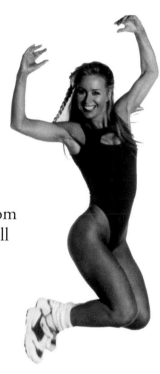

As a former patient and convert to his methods, I strongly recommend this book for everyone — from the casual walker to professional athletes. Please tell your friends about it and have fun stretching and exercising the right way for many years to come.

Best of life, lungs and leg-lifts

Cynthia Kereluk

Cynthia Kereluk is North America's #1-ranked female television exercise host. Her show "Everyday Workout" has aired internationally since 1985. This former Miss Canada has a degree in education from Simon Fraser University.

TABLE OF CONTENTS ....

Section 1   Structure: How we are designed

Function: How muscles produce motion

Stretches: Definition and mechanism

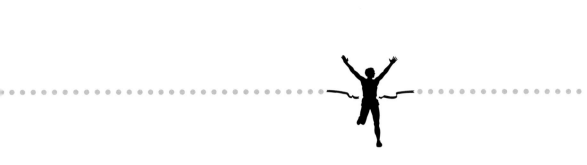

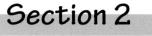

Section 3   Primary Stretches for the Major Weight-Bearing Muscle Groups of the Lower Extremity

Chapter 14   113 – 124

Groin Muscles (Adductors)

Chapter 15   125 – 134

Quadriceps

Chapter 16   135 – 152

Hamstrings

Chapter 17   153 – 166

Posterior Hip Muscles (Gluteus Maximus and the External Hip Rotators)

Chapter 18   167–176

Hip Flexors
(Psoas and the Iliacus Muscles)

Section 4   Easy Reference to
                        Correct Stretches

INTRODUCTION

As an athlete I was always fascinated by how people moved. Watching people as they exercised and trained for a specific sport was an education in the diversity of the human body.

I found it curious that athletes with similar body appearance and muscle development often had different stride lengths and varying capabilities. I began to question why some people with fairly lean muscle development had more power than those with larger, more defined muscle groups. It appeared that athletes with larger muscles were stronger and could lift more weight, but the athlete with the leaner muscles could run faster and jump higher.

My interest in movement and function led to a career as a physician. Although I completed a three-year surgical residency program after medical school, I have since dedicated my practice to focus on prevention and healing before the need for surgery. I am now a podiatric physician specializing in sports medicine and functional control. My expertise is in the structure and function of the lower extremities.

Every day in my office I see patients who are in pain:

- Teenagers, good athletes and non-athletes alike, whose most common symptom is knee pain.

- Adults who want to be more active but can't because of chronic and slowly increasing problems such as knee pain, lowback pain, or plantar fasciitis.

- Seniors who may or may not have exercised throughout their life, and who are now suffering aches and pains which are attributed to "old age."

My interest in movement and function led to a career as a physician.
Why do so many teenagers who are basically healthy have knee pain and poor posture at such a young age?

Why do we all seem to have increasing problems with joint pain and postural changes as we get older, regardless of how hard we try to stay healthy?

The answer is revealed in the study of the human gait cycle. Studying the proper sequence of *joint motion* and *phasic muscle activity* during walking or running has led to an understanding of how *muscle imbalances* cause ligament stress and joint damage in everyone.

It also explains why so many people have these problems simply doing normal daily activities without any sports involvement.

Muscle imbalances develop because the *weight bearing muscles of the lower extremity* gradually shorten over time with *repetitive usage* and *fatigue*. These large muscles will remain shortened for the rest of our lives if stretches are not done routinely and correctly.

What to do? The answer seems obvious. Everyone should include stretches for the lower extremity muscles in their daily life. Indeed, many people do stretch faithfully. However, many of these people are stretching incorrectly. They gain no benefit, and often cause permanent damage to various structures of the body.

The tremendous growth of the fitness industry has overwhelmed us with personal trainers in the fitness clubs, articles in magazines and newspapers, TV shows and video tapes on exercise and stretching. How can we distinguish between good information and bad? Where do we find current scientific facts, not personal opinions, in plain language anyone can understand and apply?

There has been an abundance of research done on how muscles function and the differences in the structure and function of muscles, tendons, and ligaments. However, this scientific data was hard to find and usually focused on the individual structures at the MOLECULAR LEVEL. This made the information too technical to be understood and translated into practical application by the average person.

We have operating manuals for our cars, VCRs, CD players — virtually everything in our lives EXCEPT OUR BODIES.

The Stark Reality Of Stretching is a comprehensive operator's manual for the body. It provides the science, the anatomy, precise definitions, and the illustrations necessary for the proper application of that knowledge to help keep the body healthy throughout our lifetime.

The Stark Reality of Stretching provides a current and concise understanding of why we should stretch, WHAT A STRETCH IS, and of course how to stretch properly. We hope that you use this book in good health!

How To Use This Book

The book is divided into four sections:

Section 1

contains the science that is necessary to explain the differences in muscles, tendons, and ligaments. This section is vital to anyone who wishes to truly understand muscle function. Understanding muscle contractions and how a muscle elongates during a stretch at the molecular level will dispel many of the myths that we have all grown up with. Accurate definitions are essential for anyone trying to instruct other people on how to exercise and stretch without injury.

Section 2

contains a summary of related topics necessary for a total picture of proper training. Included are discussions on proper warm-up exercises, how to stretch, mistakes in stretches, and a summary of the most prevalent theories on stretching.

Section 3

is the application of the knowledge gained in Sections 1 and 2. Each major muscle group of the lower extremity is examined. The anatomy, biomechanics, and proper primary stretches are explained. Important landmarks for each muscle group are illustrated. In addition, the most common mistakes made in stretching each of these muscle groups is described, and the structures that can be damaged by these errors are illustrated.

Section 4

is a quick-reference guide to proper stretches. It provides simple instructions and illustrations for the best primary stretch of any selected muscle group.

Glossary

The glossary contains as many of the terms of anatomy, biomechanics, and function as possible in order for you to review the meaning of a term or definition without having to remember where in the book you first encountered that term.

Bibliography

Throughout the book specific references are provided in shaded text boxes. These references cite the author and the date only. For example: (Ramachandran, 1967).

For the complete reference simply find this author and date in the alphabetically listed bibliography.

Illustrations

All of the illustrations in this book are original, and are meant to highlight the important anatomical landmarks and structures, as well as demonstrate good and bad stretching positions in a manner easily understood by everyone.

SECTION 1

STRUCTURE: How we are designed
FUNCTION: How muscles produce motion
STRETCHES: Definition and mechanism

Our bodies are exquisite in design and function. Every structure in our bodies is customized for a specific purpose. For example, the knee joint bends (flexes) and straightens (extends) to make our legs more mobile. The muscles whose tendons cross the knee joint produce the motion across the joint. The ligaments stabilize the joint and prevent the joint from being dislocated or injured by abnormal motion.

Proper stretching allows maximum benefits for both health and performance. This reduces the risk of potentially painful and debilitating injury to muscle and connective tissue. Stretching requires an understanding of the body structure and how it functions.

The Stark Reality of Stretching deals exclusively with the structures of the lower extremities. The following topics will be discussed with the aid of illustrations.

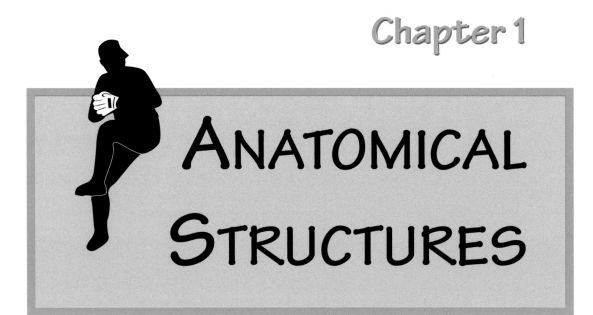

Chapter 1

ANATOMICAL STRUCTURES

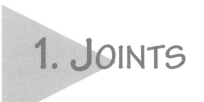

1. JOINTS

Essentially, there are three types of joints:

1. Extremely stable and virtually immovable joints, like the cranium.
2. Slightly movable joints, like the sacroiliac joint.
3. Freely movable or synovial joints, like the knee and ankle.

The joints of the lower extremities are: the hip, knee, ankle, and the many joints of the foot. All of these joints are synovial joints.

A. Definition

Joints are places of union or junction between two bones to allow motion. The two bones are joined together by ligaments, and there is articular cartilage between the bones to provide the smooth surface to allow gliding motion.

B. Purpose

Joints allow motion in order to provide mobility for the body.

■ Joint stability is provided by the ligaments that connect the two bones and limit abnormal motion of the joint, by the shape of the joint, and by other connective tissues such as the joint capsules.

■ Joint motion is produced by contraction of the muscles whose tendons cross that joint.

C. Potential Injuries

Stable joints, like the hips, provide limited movement whereas less stable joints, like the wrist, allow a wide range of motion. Although less stable joints are more easily damaged, all joints and their connective tissues can be harmed when they are forced beyond their normal range of motion.

II. CONNECTIVE TISSUE

Tendons, ligaments and fascia are comprised of connective tissue. Connective tissue is a mixture of collagenous and elastin fibers. Connective tissues are the fibrous cords that bind the individual body structures together. The differences in structure and function of collagen and elastin are very important. These differences are explained below.

A. Composition of Connective Tissue

Connective tissue is made up of two kinds of fibers: collagenous and elastic fibers.

- Collagenous fibers, rich in protein, are essentially *non-elastic.*
- Elastic fibers are characterized by the presence of the elastin protein. These fibers can be stretched, and when tension is relaxed will shorten again. They are combined with the more numerous collagenous fibers in varying amounts in connective tissue. The increased elasticity of specific ligaments and muscle fascia results from an increased percentage of elastin protein mixed with the collagen fibers.

The greatest proportion of tissue in tendons, ligaments, and fascia is collagenous fibers. The amount of elastin fibers in these structures varies with the purpose of the structure.

Tendons are composed almost totally of collagen fibers because they are not meant to stretch, while the muscle fascia has a higher concentration of elastin fibers so that it can elongate and contract.

As a person grows older, the elasticity of the connective tissue tends to deteriorate. This tendency is accelerated by inactivity, *postural malalignment and muscular imbalance.*

B. Types of Connective Tissue

(a) Tendons

Definition and Purpose

Tendons are the most inelastic connective tissue in the body. They are the tough connective tissue that attach muscle to bone. All muscles have a tendon of origin (where they originate from a bone) and a tendon of insertion (where the other end attaches by tendon to bone). The tendon of origin is usually attached to the more stable bone, while the tendon of insertion is attached to the more moveable bone.

Tendons consist almost entirely of heavy, inelastic collagen fibers that are stronger than both the muscle and the bone covering (periosteum) that the tendon attaches to.

Potential Injuries TENDONS

Tendons can be partially torn or completely ruptured if loaded beyond their tensile strength. However, since the tendon has a higher tensile strength than the muscle or the bone covering (periosteum), most excessive loads on the tendon result in tearing of the muscle tissue or the periosteum of the bone.

This means that **TENDON CANNOT BE STRETCHED.** Composed of inelastic collagen fibers, a weight of ten thousand times the molecular weight of the tendon will not stretch the tendon (Verzar, 1963).

Research indicates that microscopic fibers of tendons can be stretched to a maximum of approximately 10% of their original length before they rupture. However, at the molecular level, the fibers (protofibrils) of the tendon undergo an extension of only about 3% (Ramachandran, 1967).

In another study, a stretch of 4% was significant and corresponds to the limit of reversibility, and therefore of elasticity. At this point, the tendon's surface waviness disappears, and if the stretch continues injury may result (Crisp, 1972)

Acute Injury TENDONS

The healthy tendon will not rupture with a major overload. Instead, the muscle belly will tear or rupture and separate from the tendon; and the tendon may tear the periosteum of the bone the tendon is attached to.

A classic example of this major overload is tearing the patella tendon (tendon avulsion) completely off the front of the shin bone (the tibial tuberosity) while jumping. Several NFL football players and NBA basketball players have suffered this type of functional injury.

Chronic Injury TENDONS

Overstretching of muscle places a heavy load on the tendon. Since the tendon is inelastic (the maximum increase in length of the actual fibers of the tendon can only be 3 – 4%), what often results is a microscopic tearing of the muscle tissue or of the bone covering (periosteum).

The most common cause of damage and degeneration of tendons is extended stress due to postural faults, poor biomechanics, extended overuse, and *excessive tightness in the muscle of that tendon.*

(b) Ligaments

Definition and Purpose

Ligaments are tough connective tissues that stabilize and reinforce joints by connecting bone to bone. They consist of almost pure collagenous fiber. The amount of elasticity is again determined by the amount of elastin protein the ligaments contain.

The ligaments of the spine and the foot contain the most elastin content, which is why they are the most elastic ligaments in the body. They are therefore the easiest to damage with over-extension.

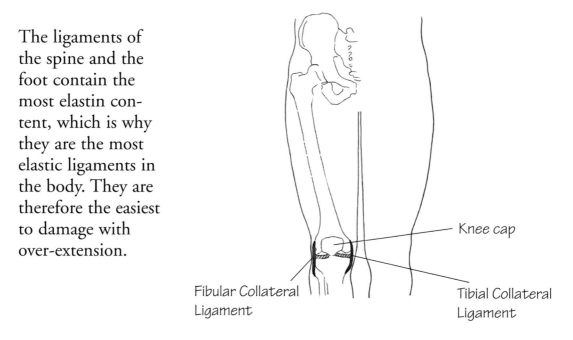

Collateral Ligaments of the Knee

The degree of elasticity in ligaments also varies with gender (in general, women have more ligament elasticity than men), age, and the level of physical fitness.

Potential Injuries LIGAMENTS

Although they are pliant and flexible, nearly all ligaments lose their ability to perform correctly when they are elongated by chronic over-extension. This is explained by the elastic and plastic properties of ligaments.

Elastic Deformity LIGAMENTS
from Acute Overload

When a joint is forced into an abnormal position during movement, the ligament has an abnormal stress applied to it. The ligament can withstand enormous forces for a very brief time. If the force is not removed, or if it exceeds the tensile strength of the ligament, then the ligament tears or ruptures. This is an elastic deformity caused by acute or sudden overload.

A classic example of this is the ankle sprain (inversion injury of the ankle). Most of these injuries are tears or complete ruptures of one or more ligaments on the lateral aspect of the ankle joint. These injuries are more severe than commonly thought, and should have immediate and proper treatment with current therapy. It takes from eight to twelve weeks to regain tensile strength in a damaged ligament, and the joint must be protected during this period with taping or with a brace.

The torn part of the ligament heals by bridging the torn fibers with scar tissue (fibrosis). The ligament will always be slightly longer and less effective in stopping abnormal joint motion, and the scar tissue will never be as strong as the original tissue. This is often the site of more tearing, chronic weakness, and repeated injury.

Plastic Deformity from Chronic Overload

When a ligament is put under a continuous and protracted stress it will gradually elongate. This is called *plastic deformity*. A classic example is the damage done to the medial collateral ligaments of the knee in the incorrect "hurdler's stretch." This is explained in the section on Hamstring stretches on page 145, Section 3.

Medial Collateral Ligament Damage

As the ligament elongates it becomes weaker, and the joint that should be stabilized by the ligament has abnormal motion (hypermobility) because the stretched ligament no longer binds the bones of the joint properly. This joint hypermobility results in chronic inflammation which may lead to degenerative arthritis.

All ligaments can be permanently elongated if subjected to protracted stress from postural faults, poor biomechanics, or *repetitive overstretching* beyond their tensile strength.

(c) Fascia

Definition and Purpose

Fascia is the connective tissue which forms enveloping sheaths around the entire muscle and each individual muscle bundle (fasciculi).

Fascia consists principally of *collagenous fibers,* although the amount of elastic fibers varies with the functional activity of the muscle. The large muscles of the extremities have a limited amount of elastic tissue.

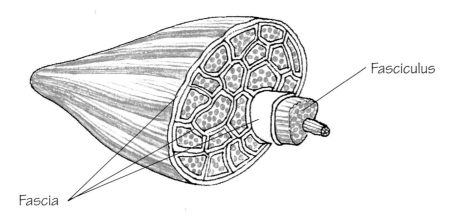

Fasciculus

Fascia

Potential Injuries

Fascia resist very high momentary tension stresses during body movement without rupturing. Protracted stress will result in permanent elongation. Fascia also has a strong tendency to shorten due to age, cold, poor posture, and *muscular imbalance.* This long-term shortening of the fascia shortens the muscle, reducing the range of motion across the joints of the body.

III. SKELETAL MUSCLE ANATOMY

There are three main types of muscle — skeletal muscle, smooth muscle (found in the internal organs) and heart muscle. In *The Stark Reality of Stretching* we are concerned with the skeletal muscles of the lower extremity: how they function, and how they stretch.

A. Definition

Skeletal muscles are the voluntary contractile tissues that move our skeletons about. They are attached directly via tendons to bones. There are more than 600 skeletal muscles in the body. These differ in size and shape according to their function.

There are six main muscle groups in the lower extremities that produce or stabilize motion:

1. the hip flexors
2. the muscles of the posterior hip (the gluteal muscles and external hip rotators)
3. the quadriceps
4. the hamstrings
5. the groin muscles (the adductors)
6. the calf muscles.

Each of these muscles or muscle groups has tendons that cross a joint. The contractions of the muscles provide the movement of the joints.

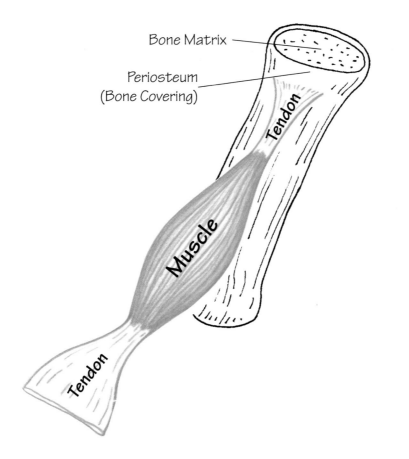

Bone Matrix

Periosteum
(Bone Covering)

Tendon

Muscle

Tendon

This diagram illustrates that all skeletal muscle originates from a tendon, and the tendon attaches to the periosteum of the bone.

B. Structure

- Muscles are made up of bundles called *fasciculi.*
- The fasciculi are made up of a group of muscle fibers composed of *myofibrils.*
- Myofibrils are made up of *sarcomeres.*
- Each Sarcomere contains two *myofilaments.*
- Myofilaments are made up of units of overlapping proteins called *myosin* and *actin.*

Myosin molecules have a long rod-shaped tail, a shorter rod-shaped neck, and two globular heads which form the cross bridges that connect to the actin protein and produce the motion required for contraction of the muscle.

The action of the cross bridging and the energy cycle of muscle contraction is important. However, the molecular level of muscle function is very technical, and beyond the scope of this book. The purpose of this book is to give athletes, coaches, everyone, an accurate understanding of muscle function and stretching that has a practical application and that translates easily when taught to others.

How muscles function, the properties of muscles, and how muscles stretch are the subjects of the next chapters.

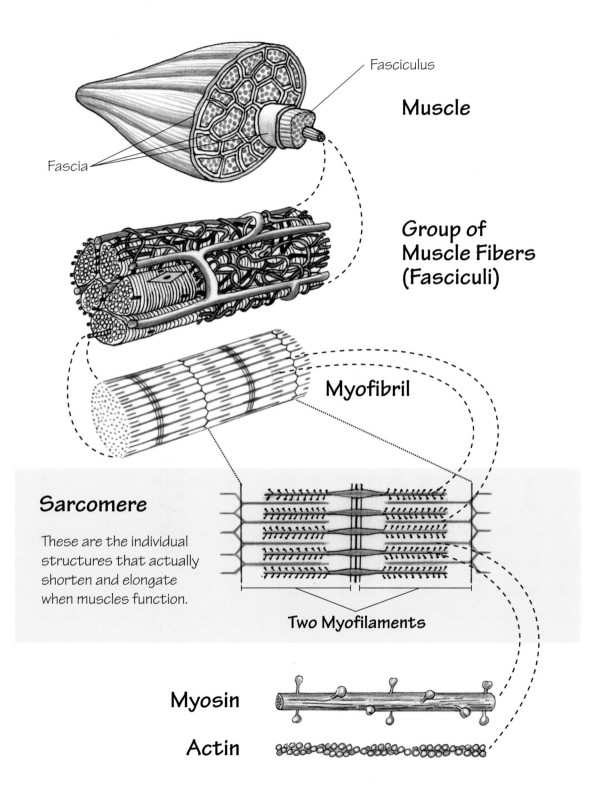

Fasciculus

Fascia

Muscle

Group of Muscle Fibers (Fasciculi)

Myofibril

Sarcomere

These are the individual structures that actually shorten and elongate when muscles function.

Two Myofilaments

Myosin

Actin

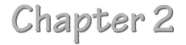

Chapter 2

HOW MUSCLES FUNCTION

Muscles shorten and elongate in order to produce motion across a joint, or they contract without changing length to hold a body position. It is important to understand the different pathways nerves can use to produce contractions of the muscle in order to appreciate what a stretch is, and how to accomplish the stretch.

Skeletal muscle contractions are either conscious *voluntary* contractions when using the muscles to lift or move an object intentionally, or *involuntary* contractions when the muscles contract in response to a loading force without conscious thought.

1. Pathways of Neuromuscular Control

A. Voluntary Contractions

When a person lifts the lower leg using the hamstring muscles, the brain (upper motor neurons) sends a message (nerve impulse) down the spinal cord to the anterior horn cells (lower motor neurons).

The lower motor neurons are the anterior and posterior horn cells of the spinal cord. They are located throughout the spinal cord wherever the large nerve roots leave the spinal cord to enter the body.

The nerve impulse then travels from the spinal cord to the muscle fibers (the motor end plates). This nerve impulse causes the hamstring muscles to contract in order to produce motion and lift the leg. This is an example of the brain directing muscle contractions to produce conscious functions.

B. Involuntary (Reflex) Contractions

When a person bends forward from the waist in a standing position, the hamstrings contract to stabilize the pelvis against gravity. If the hamstrings relaxed, the person would inevitably fall forward. The person does not think about contracting the hamstrings, and CANNOT RELAX the hamstrings while in this position.

This is an example of a reflex contraction in response
to gravity and balance; also known as a *myotactic or
proprioceptive reflex contraction.*

This reflex contraction starts with a lengthening load on the
hamstrings as the person leans forward. The nerve fibers in the
muscle (*the muscle spindles*) react to the new load and lengthening
caused by the forward bending. The muscle spindles send myotatic
nerve impulses to the spinal cord (posterior horn cells), which
direct the impulses to the anterior horn cells of the spinal cord,
which route the impulses directly back to the motor end plates of
the muscle causing an *involuntary contraction of the muscle.* This is
a "loop" of nerve cells from the muscle into the "back door" of the
spinal cord, passed on through the "front door" of the spinal cord
back to the muscles, causing them to contract.

There is no brain function (*upper motor neuron*)
involved in the initial contraction of the hamstrings
to stabilize the pelvis.

The involuntary contraction of the hamstrings
continues in order to maintain a specific postural
position against the pull of gravity. The involuntary
contraction is maintained by the myotactic reflex
caused by the proprioceptive sensors of the muscles
and brain. This becomes very important in the discussion on positioning in proper stretches.

C. Types of Contractions

All types of muscle contractions explained below can be caused by either voluntary or involuntary neuromuscular pathways.

(a) Shortening (concentric) contractions are when:

a muscle develops tension sufficient to overcome a resistance and produce work, causing the muscle to visibly shorten and move a body part against that resistance. In the individual sarcomeres of the muscles, the two myofilaments shorten by movement of the actin protein over the myosin protein toward the center of the sarcomere. This shortens the sarcomere from both ends, expends energy, and produces motion.

Sarcomeres shortening from Resting Length to Maximum Contraction

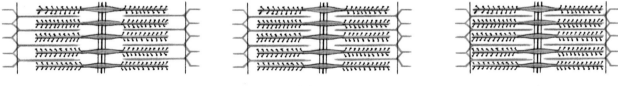

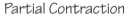

Best Resting length   Partial Contraction   Maximum Contraction

Example: When you lift your leg using the hamstring muscles, the individual sarcomeres are shortening. The muscles are shortening, expending energy and producing motion. This is a concentric contraction of the muscles.

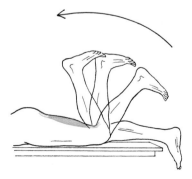

(b) Lengthening (eccentric) contractions are when:

a specific resistance or load overcomes the muscle tension and the muscle actually lengthens. In the muscles individual sarcomeres, the two myofilaments lengthen from their maximum contraction by movement of the actin protein over the myosin protein away from the center of the sarcomere. This lengthens the sarcomere at both ends, expends energy and controls motion.

Sarcomeres elongating from Maximum Contraction to Resting Length

Maximum Contraction   Partial Contraction   Best Resting length

Example: When you lower your leg using the hamstrings, the individual sarcomeres are elongating. The muscles are lengthening, expending energy and *controlling motion.* This is an eccentric contraction of the muscles.

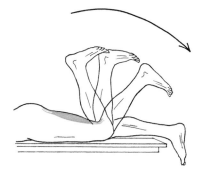

(c) Holding (isometric) contractions are when:

The muscle develops tension insufficient to move a body part against a given resistance and the length of the muscle remains unchanged. The sarcomeres are not changing length, but they are *expending energy and doing work* to maintain that position. There is no motion produced.

Sarcomeres partially contracted, expending energy, not changing length

Partial Contraction

Example: Hold the leg partially raised using the hamstring muscles to stabilize this position. The hamstrings are expending energy to maintain that position, but are not changing length. This is an isometric contraction of the muscles.

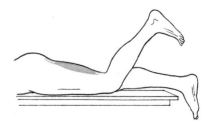

D. Resting Length

(current resting length and best resting length)

The muscle fibers are at their resting length when the muscles are not expending energy or doing work.

At their *best resting length possible* in human muscle tissue, the sarcomeres are only 25% longer than their maximally contracted length.

Sarcomere

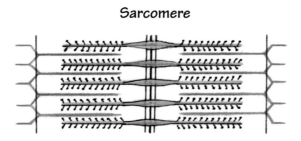

Best resting Length

The current resting length for most adults remains fairly constant in the non-weight-bearing muscles of the arms, but varies greatly in the weight-bearing muscles of the lower extremity.

For most people their current resting length is NOT their best resting length in the weight-bearing muscles of the lower extremity. This is a direct result of years of gradual shortening of the weight-bearing muscles due to repetitive motion (e.g., walking) and due to a lack of proper stretches (not extending the muscles back to the best resting length after exercise).

Most people are NOT starting their activity or sport at their best resting length. The overlapping protein fibers of weight bearing muscles have shortened in their overlap, and the surrounding connective tissue (myofascia) has shortened due to years of *not being extended back to the best resting length after exercise or repetitive motion.*

E. How Muscles Use Energy

When a muscle is doing work, it is expending energy to accomplish that work, whether the muscle is shortening, elongating, or maintaining a steady length while resisting the tension of the load placed on it.

■ Muscles expend energy and shorten to produce motion.

■ Muscles expend energy and elongate to control motion.

■ Muscles expend energy without changing length, resisting motion, in order to maintain a position.

■ Muscles store energy (e.g., during a stretch).

■ Muscles will dissipate the energy stored during a stretch as heat if the muscles are not utilized within a certain period of time after the stretch.

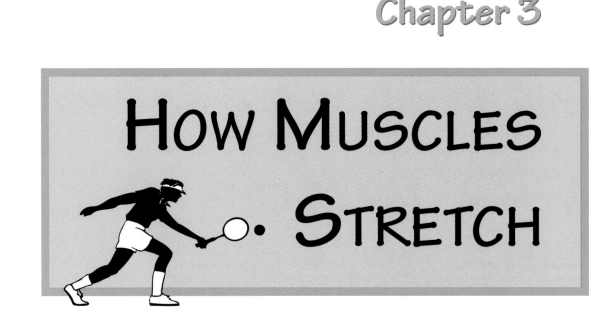

Chapter 3

HOW MUSCLES STRETCH

Unfortunately the terminology of "stretching" that we have all grown up with is misleading. When we understand the mechanisms of this muscle function, it becomes clear that nothing really stretches.

The term "stretch" leads people to think this is something they can make happen, instead of something they have to *allow* to happen.

1. DEFINITION OF A "STRETCH"

A stretch is a *sliding elongation* of the overlapping protein fibers (the actin and myosin proteins) of the myofilaments *past each other*. This results in a lengthening of the myofilaments *past their current resting length.*

The sarcomere length increases due to the elongation of the myofilaments. The myofilaments elongate because the actin and myosin protein fibers slide past each other. Neither the actin or the myosin protein fibers change length.

If a muscle or muscle group is *involuntarily contracted,* doing work and expending energy to maintain a position, the muscles cannot relax back to their resting length. The stretch, the sliding elongation of the muscle fibers past the current resting length, will never begin.

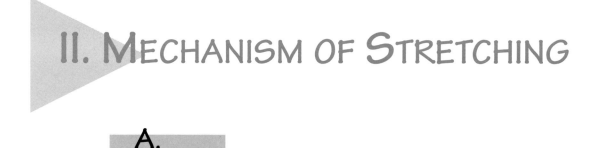

II. MECHANISM OF STRETCHING

A.

When any muscle or muscle group is initially loaded, the first thing that happens is a lower motor neuron reflex contraction. The relaxed muscles contract in response to the loading force. All of those millions of sarcomeres shorten. At this point the muscle is contracted and expending energy to resist the initial load placed on the muscle.

B.

If the tension on the muscle is held long enough, in a position where the muscles can relax (i.e., it is not expending energy to maintain that position), and if the muscle is not overloaded, the muscle's sarcomeres will relax back to their *original resting length*. The muscle is no longer expending energy to resist the gentle tension.

C.

Only then will the gentle tension left on the muscle cause the sliding elongation of the overlapping protein fibers of the sarcomeres past their resting length. As the sarcomeres lengthen they store energy. The sliding elongation of the sarcomeres continues until there is no tension left on the muscle.

A. Initial Contraction

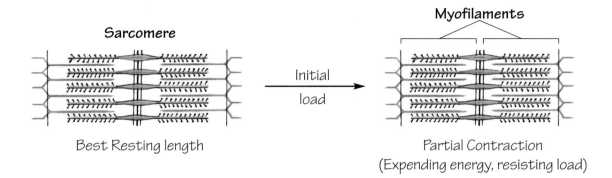

Sarcomere

Myofilaments

Initial
load

Best Resting length

Partial Contraction
(Expending energy, resisting load)

B. Relaxation

Partial Contraction

Relaxing

Best Resting length
(No longer expending energy)

C. Sliding Elongation

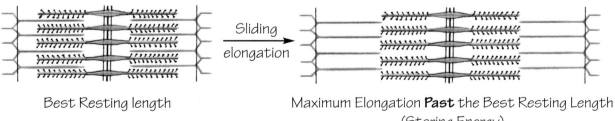

Best Resting length

Sliding
elongation

Maximum Elongation **Past** the Best Resting Length
(Storing Energy)

III. MAXIMUM LENGTH OF SARCOMERES

The myofilaments have a finite distance they can elongate through this sliding elongation. The actin protein cannot slide past the end of the myosin protein. The cross bridging must be maintained for muscle function.

Muscle fibers have a maximally contracted length, a best resting length, and a maximum elongation *past their best resting length.*

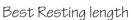

Maximum Contraction   Best Resting length   Maximum Elongation **Past**
the Best Resting Length

A maximally contracted muscle fiber (sarcomere) is approximately 25% shorter than its best resting length. At its longest possible length *after stretching* the sarcomere is *60-70% LONGER than at its best resting length.*

Chapter 4

PROPERTIES OF MUSCLES

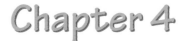

I. MUSCLE STRENGTH

Strength is defined as "contractibility, the capacity to shorten and the ability to develop tension." Through exercise the number of individual muscle fibers (sarcomeres) is increased. This increase in the mass of the muscle increases the muscle's ability to develop tension.

Strength is simply translated as how large the mass of the muscle is, how much load a muscle can *hold,* and how much *tension* the muscle can develop without tearing.

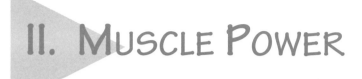

II. MUSCLE POWER

Power is defined as how much load a muscle can *move* and how *fast* that muscle can move a specific load. A muscle has its most *power* when the individual muscle fibers are at their longest length of contraction. That muscle can move a larger load at a faster speed. As the muscle fibers shorten (contract), the load they can move and/or the speed they can move that load decreases.

This is what makes stretching so vitally important to athletes!!!

Pre-stretched muscle (stretching the muscle before the sports or activity) functions with greater efficiency because elastic energy is stored in the muscle tissue during stretching and is recovered during the subsequent shortening (Asmussen & Bonde-Petersin, 1974; Boscoe, Tarkka, & Komi, 1982; Cavagna, Dusman, & Margaria, 1968; Ciullo & Zarins, 1983; Grieve, 1970; Komi & Boscoe, 1978).

The only way to *increase power* is to *elongate the muscles' sarcomeres past their current resting length prior to the sports activity.*

A muscle exerts its greatest tension when it functions at its greatest length. It can lift a greater load or produce a greater force the more it is pre-stretched from its resting length prior to contraction (Hill, A.V., 1956).

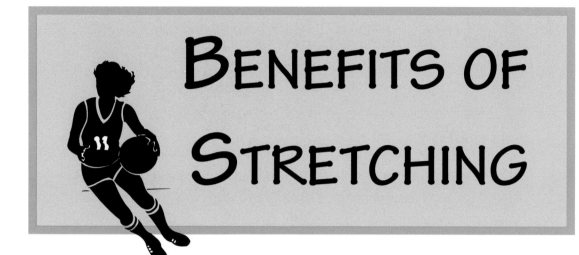

Chapter 5

BENEFITS OF STRETCHING

▶ I. BENEFITS FOR ATHLETES: PERFORMANCE

By using proper warm-ups and stretches on a consistent basis, athletes can achieve their full potential in sports and *extend their best performance* for many years.

With proper stretching they can avoid the long-term consequences of secondary muscle, ligament, and joint damage caused by muscular imbalance and training errors.

Many young athletes have their personal-best performance when they are 16 or 17 years old. At this age they are still structurally immature.

At age 20-21 these athletes should be in their prime. They are more mature in the joint structure and have more *muscle mass.* Although this gives them more strength, they are unable to run as fast or jump as high as they could when they were younger. Many of these athletes are spending up to 50% of their training year trying to recover from chronic and recurring injuries, particularly to the knee, hip, and back.

These athletes have developed more *muscle mass and strength, but have less power.* They cannot equal their personal-best performance of earlier years and are chronically injured. This is a direct result of *too much strength and skill level training* combined with *not enough or incorrect stretches.*

With all strength-training programs it is essential to incorporate a stretching program. Get the strength by increasing the muscle mass through exercise, then get the power by elongating the individual muscle fibers through stretching.

II. BENEFITS FOR CHILDREN

Growing children are especially prone to developing muscle imbalances due to their rapid growth rate. Longitudinal growth occurs in the bones, along with the soft tissues such as the muscles and tendons. It is important that all children learn to stretch properly and consistently to maintain good muscle balance, joint range of motion, and to prevent injuries.

During periods of rapid growth there can be an increase in muscle-tendon tightness about the joints and a loss of range of motion due to the bones growing much faster than the muscles lengthen. (Kendall & Kendall, 1948; Leard, 1984; Micheli, 1983; Sutro, 1947).

III. BENEFITS FOR EVERYONE

It is important for people to realize how essential stretching is as ongoing maintenance of the weight-bearing muscles. Everyone needs to maintain good symmetry and length in these muscle groups in order to stay healthy and active.

A. Benefits of Maintaining Proper Muscle Length and Symmetry in the Lower Extremity

Muscle shortening will gradually change everyone's joint position and stride length. This in turn causes much of the chronic, insidious damage to the ligaments, which results in changes in joint position and posture.

> Many people think that the chronic ache in their knees and lowback as they age is inevitable. "Rheumatism" is still a term often heard in discussions with elderly people.

Except for people with an underlying systemic disease such as rheumatoid arthritis, this is not true. Most of the chronic, low-level inflammation and pain in their muscles and joints is the result of *how they function, not how old they are.*

Most of these people can be helped by correcting the structural and muscle imbalances of their lower extremity through stretching. Better muscle function, joint position, and stride length will reduce the stress on their ligaments and joints.

No one has identified the problem and taught the older athlete how to change the muscle function that is causing the joint damage and postural changes (Corbin & Noble, 1980). Present medical treatment is all too often focused on the *symptom* instead of the *cause*.

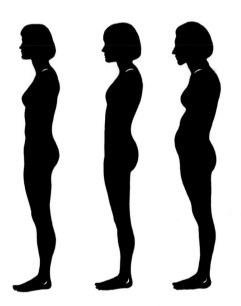

Posture changes with aging because of ligament stretching and changes in joint position. *This does not have to happen!*

Postural Changes with Ageing

B. Benefits from Relaxation of Muscle

Habitually tense muscles tend to reduce their own circulation. Reduced blood supply results in a lack of oxygen and essential nutrients and causes toxic waste products to accumulate in the cells. *This will cause fatigue, aches, even pain.*

Relaxation is an economical energy consumption and resistance to fatigue (Basmajian, 1975). When more muscle fibers than necessary are activated, an inefficient energy expenditure results (Coville, 1979).

Relaxation of the muscles is a valuable part of stretching. Excessive muscular tension tends to decrease sensory awareness and raise blood pressure (Larson & Michelman, 1973).

IV. PREVENTION OF INJURIES

When exercising to stimulate muscle growth (increase muscle mass), the length of the individual muscle fibers are shortened by the repetitive usage and fatigue. Over a prolonged period of time this muscle shortening can cause muscle imbalances that lead to ligament damage, joint hypermobility, and loss of function and power.

Stretching helps prevent injuries by not allowing the gradual, insidious shortening of the individual muscle fibers caused by repetitive usage and fatigue. The more the muscles are used, the more maintenance they require. *That maintenance is stretching.*

Chapter 6

SUMMARY

■ Muscles are the contractile tissue that produce and control motion across the joints.

■ A sarcomere is the individual muscle fiber containing two myofilaments.

■ The myofilaments contain the actin and myosin protein fibers. It is the actin and myosin protein fibers sliding back and forth past each other that expend energy and produce motion. *The two myofilaments of each sarcomere are the contractile tissues of the muscle that produce contractions.*

■ A sarcomere has a resting length, where the muscle is not expending energy or doing work.

SUMMARY

■ A sarcomere has a maximum contraction, where the protein overlap cannot shorten any further. The sarcomere length cannot shorten past that point.

■ *All movement and exercise* takes place somewhere between a muscle fibers' *current resting length* and it's *maximum contraction.*

■ *STRENGTH* is defined as contractibility, the capacity to shorten and the ability to develop tension. Exercise increases the number of individual muscle fibers (sarcomeres), increasing the muscle mass. The larger the muscle mass, the more tension the muscle can develop.

■ *POWER* is defined as how much load a muscle can move and how fast that muscle can move a specific load. Power comes from the longest length of contraction possible in the *individual muscle fibers* (sarcomeres).

■ The only way to elongate the muscle fibers past the current resting length and gain more power is *through proper stretches.*

■ A stretch is a sliding elongation of the overlapping protein fibers of the myofilaments *past their current resting length.* This results in an elongation of the sarcomeres.

■ *ENERGY* is stored in the muscle during this sliding elongation, giving the muscle more *POWER.*

SUMMARY

- The non-weight-bearing muscles of the arms will have approximately the same resting length throughout a lifetime. They simply are not functioning under the constant and enormous load of the weight-bearing muscles of the lower extremity.

- The weight-bearing muscles of the lower extremity will slowly shorten in their resting length over the years with repetitive usage, even without sports involvement. The *current resting length* is very seldom the *best resting length* in these muscles.

- These muscles will remain shortened and asymmetrical if the person does not learn the importance of stretching, and how to do proper stretches.

- In athletes, this gradual shortening will affect their performance levels as well as lead to chronic injuries.

- In everyone, the shortening of the lower extremity muscles will lead to changes in joint position and stride length in all walking functions. This will always lead to gradual ligament damage, causing changes in joint position and posture.

- Stretching of the weight-bearing muscle groups of the lower extremity is the body maintenance that we need throughout life. With proper stretching we can achieve better function and more power; and avoid many of the long-term problems such as arthritis, muscle stiffness and chronic discomfort that affect so many people.

Notes

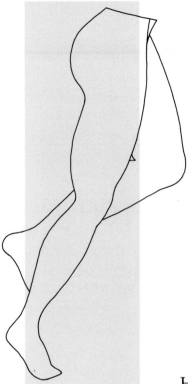

SECTION 2

Muscle Preparation
How to Stretch
Mistakes in Stretching

Having discussed muscle anatomy and the mechanisms of the muscle myofilament elongation during a "stretch," we now need to know how to make this knowledge practical for everyone. Before the proper stretch for each of the weight-bearing muscle groups is described, several related topics must be examined.

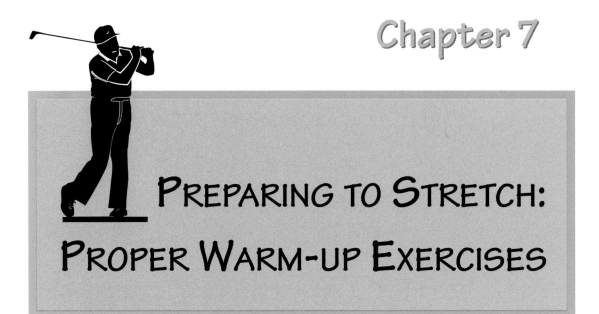

PREPARING TO STRETCH: PROPER WARM-UP EXERCISES

The terms warm-ups and stretches are often confused. Warm-up exercises are not stretches. In order to prevent injury to the muscles it is important to do warm-up exercises as a *preparation* for stretches.

I. DEFINITION

Warm-ups are not stretches. Warm-ups are *gentle* exercises done to prepare the muscles for stretching.

■ Cold muscle has a poor blood supply, a high viscosity (meaning it has a high chemical *inelasticity*), and therefore can be easily injured by stretching without doing proper warm-up exercises first.

■ Warm-up exercises are defined as repetitive contractions of the muscles under a light to moderate load, in order to literally increase the heat (warmth, blood flow) of the muscles. During these repetitive gentle contractions the blood flow increases, and the viscosity of the muscle decreases (the elasticity of the muscle increases).

Stretches should always be *preceded* by a mild set of warm-up exercises. The increase in the tissue temperature and blood flow produced by the muscular exercise will make the stretching both safer and more productive (Sapega et al., 1981).

CHAPTER 7

II. TYPES OF WARM-UPS

A. Walking

A classic example of a gentle, repetitive contraction is walking. WALKING is an ideal warm-up exercise. A five-minute walk is a good warm-up. A ten-minute walk is an exemplary warm-up. While walking the muscles of the upper and lower extremities, especially the five major weight-bearing muscle groups of the lower extremity, are going through repetitive gentle contractions. These repetitive contractions under a light load increase the blood flow and elasticity of the muscles. It is important to understand that the *weight-bearing impact* of walking is *three to four times less* than running or jumping.

B. Gentle Power Movements with Light Weights

Using light weights in weight training has been recommended as warm-up exercises for specific muscle groups in some research.

The purpose of warming up is to raise the internal temperature and reduce the viscosity in the muscles. The Russians have found that including preliminary strength-training exercises for the hamstring muscles in their warm-ups prevents rupture of the muscle fibers.

Volkov and Mironova studied the temperature of the thigh (femoral) muscles and observed a *decrease* in the temperature of these muscles during common but incorrect warm-up exercises. After inclusion of power exercises for the hamstrings at the beginning of the warm-up, an increase of 1.6 to 2.6 degrees (centigrade) was recorded in the muscles internal temperature (Volkov, M.V. & Mironova, Z.S., 1966).

C. Other Warm-up Exercises

Other exercises such as cycling, treadmill, and rowing at moderate loads are also good warm-up exercises.

III. INCORRECT WARM-UPS

There are many examples of incorrect warm-up exercises, including *running slowly* and *jumping rope,* which often lead to injury.

To understand why running slowly to warm up is a training error, we need to understand how the body absorbs the shock of the landing impact through muscle function; and how the body spreads (*dissipates*) that shock over the largest surface area of the joints. There are three important factors involved in the *mechanisms of shock absorption* and the *dissipation of that shock* in walking and running.

IV. MECHANISMS OF SHOCK ABSORPTION

A. Muscle Function

B. Joint Range of Motion

C. Horizontal Displacement of the Body Mass

A. Muscle Function

The lower extremity muscles, elongating and shortening in stride (eccentric and concentric muscle contractions), absorb most of the shock of the landing impact. Muscle function is the number-one *"shock absorber"* of the body.

Description of Shock Absorption by the Lower Leg Muscles:

The lower leg muscles, whose tendons extend into the foot, absorb shock. These muscle groups must elongate and expend energy (an eccentric contraction) to decelerate the forefoot impact and absorb shock all the way through pronation (the first stage of the midstance phase of gait in everyone).

Cold muscles cannot elongate under load (eccentrically contract) effectively, because the muscles do not have good blood flow or elasticity. The sudden ballistic loading of the landing impact causes thousands of microtears at the muscle-tendon junctions of both the anterior and deep posterior muscle groups of the lower leg.

SHOCK ABSORPTION

- This chronic tearing of tissue causes the pain and pressure from swelling (edema) in *shin splints*.

- If enough tissue is torn to have serious swelling and increased pressure in the surrounding fascial compartment, it is referred to as a *compartment syndrome*.

- Because these muscles are not absorbing shock and the bone is trying to reorganize and increase its calcium density to handle the increased shock, this often results in a *tibial* or *metatarsal stress fracture*.

One of the most common causes of shin splints, compartment syndromes and stress fractures is a very simple training error: *running slowly to warm up*. By the time the athlete is clinically symptomatic, the microscopic tearing has been occurring for a prolonged period of time.

B. Joint Range of Motion

The next important component of the body's ability to handle the shock of the landing impact is joint range of motion. The longer the stride, the larger the range of motion (of the foot, ankle, knee, and hip joints). This spreads the shock over the largest articular surface area of each joint. There is *less impact* on any given part of the cartilage of each joint. Spreading the landing impact over a larger area of the articular cartilage of the joint diminishes the shock on that joint.

C. Horizontal Displacement of the Body Mass

The more horizontal momentum of the body mass, parallel to the ground, the less vertical vector force into the ground. In other words, the better the horizontal momentum, the less impact when the foot strikes the ground (see example next page).

SHOCK ABSORPTION

Example:

The following example demonstrates how these three factors affect shock absorption.

> A 200-lb. man walking at a steady pace with good muscle function, joint position, and stride length, will hit the ground with his body weight plus approximately 20% (which amounts to about *240 lb./sq. in. of loading force* as his foot impacts on the ground).

The same 200 lb. man running well, not sprinting *but not jogging slowly,* has almost the identical muscle function and joint range of motion as he had walking, but with a longer stride length. He maintains good horizontal momentum of his body mass but *significantly increases his velocity,* which will triple the weight-bearing impact into the ground. The *momentum of impact* is now approximately *720 lb./ sq. in.* while running at a decent stride length, and *he is still maximizing the body's ability to absorb and dissipate that shock.*

> Jogging slowly shortens the stride, *reducing the joint range of motion* and decreasing muscle function. The body's ability to absorb and dissipate shock has been decreased. The slow runner also loses or greatly reduces the horizontal momentum, therefore *the*

SHOCK ABSORPTION

vertical vector force is increased. He has reduced his body's ability to handle impact while increasing the impact in comparison to walking. Running slowly, he as at least doubled his impact to approximately 480 lb./sq. inch. Running slowly **to warm-up,** on cold lower leg muscles that have reduced blood flow and limited eccentric capacity, is a major cause of many "over-use" injuries.

V. SUMMARY

By studying the physics of motion and the momentum of impact, it is obvious that running slowly has a higher impact than when walking at a fast pace; and the body has less ability to absorb and dissipate shock. Running slowly to warm-up is a training error.

Because of the increased joint trauma, running slowly over long periods of time on hard surfaces can cause degenerative changes of the foot, knee, hip, pelvis, and spine in anyone.

THE SOLUTION IS SIMPLE!!!

Everyone who runs or jumps in their sports should **WALK** for at least five minutes as a **WARM-UP!!** You take several hundred steps in a five-minute walk. This allows the lower leg muscles multiple contractions with 2-3 times less impact than running. The muscle's blood flow increases, the viscosity decreases, and their ability to eccentrically contract is greatly enhanced.

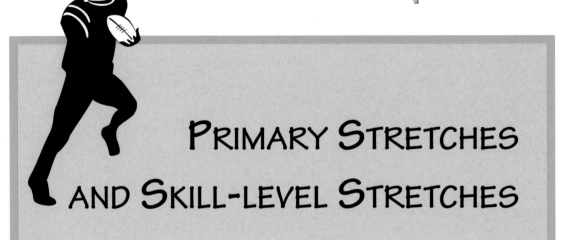

Chapter 8

PRIMARY STRETCHES AND SKILL-LEVEL STRETCHES

There are two levels of stretches. Everyone needs to do primary stretches for health and well-being. Only athletes, who are doing movements that require an extremely large range of motion across their joints, should be doing skill-level stretches.

I. PRIMARY STRETCHES

Primary stretches isolate one major muscle or muscle group across one joint, in a position where the muscle group can relax back to its resting length and slide longer. Structures such as the ligaments of the joints or the joint capsules are not loaded if the

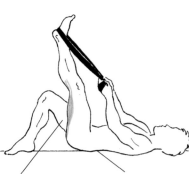

stretch is done with proper positioning. Important structures like the sciatic nerve in the posterior pelvis are not put under any traction which could result in damage.

Isolates the Hamstring Muscles

No Load on Pelvic or Spinal Ligaments

II. SKILL-LEVEL STRETCHES

Skill-level stretches load more than one major muscle group, and place a heavy load on other structures of the body, especially the ligaments of the pelvis and spine. They should only be done *after* the individual muscle groups have stretched to their maximum length in a primary stretch, and only after years of training beginning at an early age.

The ligaments of the body have the most elasticity during early puberty and adolescence. Growth hormones allow ligaments to elongate without tearing in order to keep up with the rapid growth of the bones. If the ligament elongation was not able to keep pace with the rapid growth of the bones at this age, everyone would suffer some ligament tearing and damage. Stretches that place a large load on the ligaments must be learned at this time of life, and continued through the adult years.

Because the growth hormone is no longer present in adults, anyone trying to start these skill-level stretches as adults will suffer tearing and damage to the ligaments.

Loading Pelvis and Lumbar Ligaments

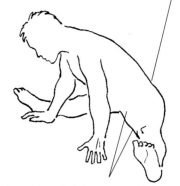

Loading Adductor and Medial Hamstring Muscles

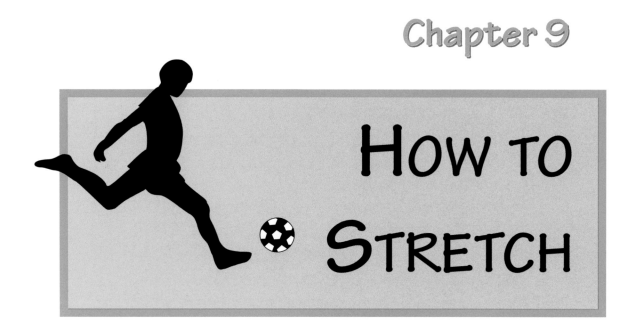

Chapter 9

HOW TO STRETCH

After careful consideration of the published literature of the last sixty years, and my experiences both as an amateur and professional athlete, followed by years as a physician specializing in sports medicine, I have come to this conclusion:

For the majority of people, whether active athletes or those trying to stay healthy, stretching is of vital importance. In order to accomplish their stretches and not cause damage to the muscles or other structures, certain criteria must be met in terms of positioning and which specific structures are loaded. The following are the criteria for proper static stretches.

1. The stretch must be simple and can be accomplished by *one individual* without the aid of a partner.

2. The stretch must isolate *one major muscle* or *muscle group* of the lower extremity in a position where that muscle group can relax back to its resting length and slide longer.

3. With proper positioning and isolation of one specific muscle group other structures such as ligaments and the sciatic nerve are not loaded to any significant level.

4. When stretching before any athletic activity, I recommend that each muscle group be stretched twice in succession. The way to accomplish this is to find the first tension and wait for that tension to release, then find that same gentle tension a second time and allow the muscle to elongate again.

DISCUSSION

Discussion of Criteria 4:

■ When the muscle group is loaded gently, the muscle fibers relax back to their current resting length fairly quickly, and the sliding elongation then occurs. This is experienced as a loss of sensation (tension).

  ■ Because the muscles are being loaded gently, there is not enough tension to cause the muscle fibers to slide a great distance. Once the first tension is gone, find that gentle tension again; and allow the second loss of sensation (tension).

■ The muscle fibers are now *two segments longer* in their myofilaments than before the initial stretch.

  ■ Sometimes it is possible to do three segments of stretching on a muscle group, although often the tension you feel in the third segment does not decrease. This is because the myofilaments have reached their longest possible length. The actin protein cannot slide past the last cross-link with the myosin protein, or the myofilament would tear.

You now have the most power from the longest length of contraction possible!

Breathing enhances stretching:

Controlled breathing not only facilitates relaxation, it also enhances stretching (Jencks, 1977). Stretching is enhanced by exhalation. Inhaling slowly and deeply, followed by exhaling slowly and completely, will facilitate the muscles' relaxation and elongation past their current resting length.

Chapter 10

THE 5 GOLDEN RULES OF STRETCHING

The five golden rules of stretching are stated below. These rules apply to any major muscle group, and incorporate the information contained in the previous chapters. By following these simple guidelines many benefits are gained, including better symmetry, length, and power in your muscles.

Isolate the Muscle Group

- Isolate the muscle group across one joint in a position where the muscle group is not expending energy to maintain that position.
- The positioning of the muscle group should not load other structures such as ligaments or joint capsules.

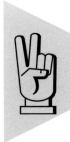

Find Zero Tension

- Zero tension is when there is *no awareness of tension* in a muscle group because there is no load and resulting tension on that muscle group.
- When you start with *no tension* in the muscle group and then find the first tension or awareness, the biofeedback of that muscle group is more subtle and accurate.
- When you start a stretch with tension in the muscle group and try to adjust the tension on that muscle group, the biofeedback is not as subtle or accurate.

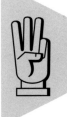

Find the First Awareness

- Find the first gentle tension in the muscle group *(the gentle reflex contraction against the loading force)*. This is the first awareness of a stretch.
- Loading the muscles harder serves no purpose! It will take longer for the muscles to relax back to their original resting length. The sliding elongation of the overlapping protein fibers past the original resting length *does not start* until that relaxation has occurred.
- By loading the muscles harder the desired effect is delayed and there is more risk of injury due to overstretching.
- This leads us to Rule #4.

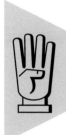

Less is Best

- As just explained, the more gentle the initial load on a muscle or muscle group in a stretch, the faster the muscle group can relax back to the current resting length.
- The muscle group must relax back to the *current resting length* before the sliding elongation past the resting length can begin.

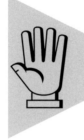

Allow the Loss of Tension

- Stretches *cannot* be timed. The gentle tension must be steady and constant on the muscle if the muscle fibers are going to relax and slide past their current resting length.
- The duration of a stretch changes daily. It is determined by many factors:
  - The amount of initial load on the muscle group.
  - The amount of warm-up before the stretch.
  - The fatigue in the muscle, or any inflammation from injury or overuse.
- Find the first gentle tension in the muscle group and maintain a steady position until the tension is gone.
- *Allow* the muscles the time required for the relaxation/elongation. *You cannot make it happen.* Do not watch the clock. Listen to your body and depend on your biofeedback.

BIOFEEDBACK

Biofeedback is the body awareness *developed* through movement, exercise, and stretches. Most people have been taught to stretch with intensity or pain in the muscles ("No Pain, No Gain" has been the maxim). Their biofeedback has been conditioned to intensity.

Initially these people may have trouble feeling the gentle tension of a proper stretch. This will change with proper stretching techniques and practice. Learning to find the first gentle tension in the muscles will result in better and more subtle biofeedback.

MISTAKES IN STRETCHING

Many young athletes and people in fitness programs are causing themselves long-term damage instead of benefiting from their participation because of training errors.

Older athletes are far more crippled by the *muscle imbalances, ligament weakening, joint hypermobility,* and the *resulting joint damage* caused by these training errors over a lifetime than by all of the acute injuries they have experienced.

Common mistakes in stretching are due to:
- Timing
- Positioning errors
- Loading other structures
- Overstretching

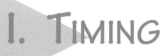 **I.** TIMING

Timing relates to two aspects of stretching:

A. How long to hold a stretch

People are taught that a stretch can be timed. "Hold that stretch for thirty seconds" is a common recommendation. This is *incorrect. No one can time stretches.*

> When loading a muscle, the relaxation time back to the original resting length will vary greatly from individual to individual.

The relaxation time is directly related to how much load is initially placed on the muscles. The harder you load a muscle group, the longer it takes for the muscles to relax.

> It will also vary in the same person from day to day because of fatigue. A tired muscle is shorter and chemically more inelastic. It will have a much longer relaxation time than the same muscle the day it is rested.

The timing of a stretch is determined by holding the position until the tension in the muscle group is gone.

B. When to stretch
(the time lapse between the
stretch and the competition)

A stretch should *immediately precede* the skill-level activity or sports competition in order for the athlete to take advantage of the increased power of the muscles.

If a sprinter warms up and stretches, then stands around for 20-30 minutes before the competition, the muscles will contract back to their original resting length. *As a result, the energy stored in the muscles by stretching is WASTED.*

If a muscle is not used after stretching, relaxation back toward its current resting length will occur. The energy stored in the stretching is not taken advantage of and the stored elastic energy is dissipated as heat (Hill, 1961).

II. POSITIONING

The muscle or muscle group must be isolated in a position *where the muscles are not contracted or expending energy* to maintain that position or posture.

There are many examples of incorrect stretching positions where the muscle group is *involuntarily contracted* to stabilize the body against gravity. All standing hamstring muscle stretches are an example of this positioning error. These are described in detail in Section 3.

III. LOADING OTHER STRUCTURES

Primary stretches isolate one muscle group across one joint, without loading other structures unrelated or connected to this specific muscle group or joint.

There are many examples of loading other structures and the damage that can occur to ligaments, joint capsules, and the sciatic nerve as a result. These will be discussed in detail as each muscle group is described in Section 3.

Improper positioning resulting in ligament damage is illustrated in this example.

When a ligament is put under a continuous and protracted stress it will gradually elongate.

As described in the section on the different properties of connective tissue, ligaments in adults can only elongate through a process of *microscopic tearing, scarring, and weakening.* This is call *plastic deformity.*

The weakened and elongated ligaments are no longer able to stabilize the bones of the joint properly, which results in hypermobility of the joint. This excessive joint motion causes joint trauma and chronic inflammation. The chronic inflammation results in the gradual destruction of the joint cartilage. This destruction of the joint cartilage is called degenerative arthritis (osteoarthritis).

Any stretch that loads the joints and places an abnormal stress on the ligaments will slowly cause permanent damage to the ligaments. The so-called "hurdler's stretch" is a classic example. In stretching the hamstrings of one leg, the ligaments of the opposite knee are placed under abnormal stress.

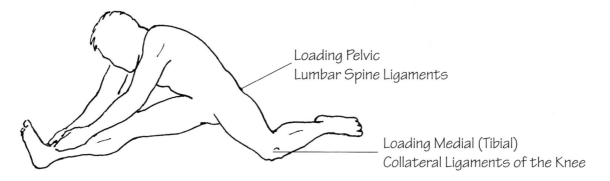

Loading Pelvic
Lumbar Spine Ligaments

Loading Medial (Tibial)
Collateral Ligaments of the Knee

When the knee is flexed and externally rotated in this *weight-bearing* position there is an abnormal load placed on the medial collateral ligaments of the knee. Flexion of the knee joint in this position will damage the ligaments (Rapoport, 1984; Anderson, 1980).

When this is done repetitively over a long period of time, the end result is the tearing, scarring, and weakening of the ligaments of the bent knee, as the athlete tries to stretch the hamstrings of the other leg.

IV. OVERSTRETCHING

Overstretching is placing too much tension on a muscle group, causing damage to the muscle fibers.

Overstretching causes microscopic tearing at the muscle-tendon junctions, the weakest part of any muscle, and causes permanent scarring (fibrosis) in the muscle fibers. With a major overload, the tendon attachment to the bone can be torn, especially in children. *Remember, the tendon fibers cannot elongate more than 3-4% without rupturing the tendon.*

The problem with overstretching is that it does not hurt during the stretch. People feel the contraction and pull in the wrong place, but don't feel pain. The resulting microscopic tearing is not sufficient to cause *immediate* inflammation in the structures. The *minor soreness* at the ends of the muscles is usually more apparent the *next day.*

Knowing where to feel the tension during a stretch, AND WHERE NOT TO FEEL ANY TENSION, is very important. When viewing the illustrations of each muscle group in Section 3 this is easily understood.

Examples:

■ You should never feel any tension up to or behind the knee when doing calf stretches. The upper muscle-tendon junction of the gastrocnemius muscle is just below the knee joint. There is very little gastrocnemius muscle behind the knee, only *joint capsule* and the gastrocnemius muscle's tendon of origin.

■ You should not feel any tension from a hand's width above the knee down to the knee when doing hamstring stretches. The hamstring's muscle-tendon junction is 4-8 inches above the knee. When the tension of the stretch is felt behind the knee, there is no immediate sensation of pain.

■ When the muscle is crampy and sore at the ends of the muscles (tendon junctions) *the next day,* you don't realize that the stretch the day before has caused the damage.

V. GOOD SORENESS/BAD SORENESS

How do you know when you are making mistakes while stretching? The microscopic tearing caused by overstretching does not cause immediate inflammation and pain. It often takes 12-24 hours for the inflammation and minor discomfort caused by that tearing to become obvious.

Because you usually do not register pain when overstretching, you need to become aware of the body's signals the next day. Body awareness the next day will help you to learn the difference between good soreness and bad soreness.

A. Good Soreness

When muscles are exercised to fatigue (anaerobic metabolism), they will be sore and stiff *throughout the entire muscle* the next morning. After hours of movement, with increased blood flow and lymphatic drainage, this morning soreness gradually disappears.

This is the *good soreness* of endurance or strength training. The explanation for this soreness is varied in the literature.

GOOD SORENESS

The accumulation of lactic acid, the excessive accumulation of metabolites that cause an increased osmotic pressure inside and outside muscle fiber, retained excess water causing edema and pressure on sensory nerves are just a few of the current theories (Asmussen, 1956; Karpovich & Sinning, 1971).

Others feel that the swelling of the muscle tissue with the accumulation of metabolites causes the muscle to become shorter, thicker, and more resistant to stretching or movement. This is what causes the sensation of stiffness (Morehouse & Miller, 1971).

The old and inaccurate theory that muscle soreness is due to microscopic tearing of the muscle fibers and connective tissue (Hough, 1902) is incorrect. It is not sensible or plausible to think that a tissue is structurally damaged by the function for which it is specifically differentiated (de Vries, 1961a, 1961b, 1962, 1966).

B. Bad Soreness

If the good soreness goes away, and there is pain or obvious discomfort at the end of the muscle, or in the ligaments or joint capsules, this is the *bad soreness caused by training errors.*

This bad soreness of microscopic tearing and scarring can last for days or weeks; and in some cases last the entire training year.

It is imperative to teach people simple landmarks of muscle anatomy, and to teach the difference between good soreness and bad soreness.

Summary:

By learning simple landmarks of the body and understanding the concept of good soreness/bad soreness, you can recognize and eliminate training errors and the resulting injuries.

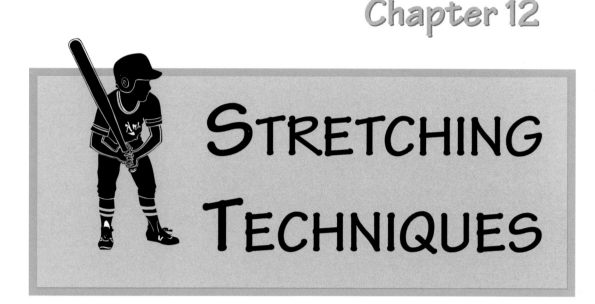

Chapter 12

STRETCHING TECHNIQUES

There has been a lot of research concerning how muscles function, and what is the best method of stretching. Everyone in sports seems to have a different theory on this topic.

The following is a brief review of some of these stretching techniques. When studied closely, some of the stretching techniques do not make sense when the mechanisms of stretching are understood. Other techniques, like PNF stretching, require a thorough knowledge of neuromuscular function and a well-trained partner.

1. DYNAMIC STRETCHES

Dynamic stretches, also called active extensions, are not stretches *by definition.* The muscles are isometrically contracting to maintain the position. As previously discussed, *this is not a stretch* because the muscles cannot relax back to their current resting length; therefore no sliding elongation past the current resting length can occur.

A classic example of a dynamic contraction is the runner's "stretch."

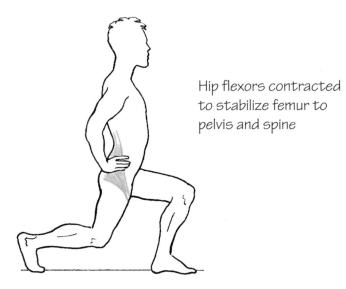

Hip flexors contracted to stabilize femur to pelvis and spine

Although dynamic extensions are not stretches, they are *good mobilization exercises,* and will help maintain healthy sarcomeres at the ends of the muscles.

Muscles that have been shortened by injury or lack of use lose the sarcomeres at the ends of the muscle. One study showed a 40% loss of sarcomeres in series with prolonged contracture (Tabary et al., 1972).

Muscles that are *continually placed in an extended position* can regenerate sarcomeres in series at the ends of the muscle. This is why dynamic extensions and end of range of motion exercises are beneficial. There should never be any ballistic or bouncing motions to these mobilization exercises.

II. PNF STRETCHES

One of the most often discussed forms of stretching is the PNF method. PNF stands for *Proprioceptive Neuromuscular Facilitation.* How many people can pronounce this, much less know what it means or how to accomplish it effectively without causing damage?

Two people are required for most PNF stretches. The technique requires the person stretching to contract the muscle group being stretched against resistance from the partner. Then the *opposite muscle group* is contracted while tension to the muscle group being stretched is applied by the partner. The opposite muscle group must remain consciously contracted while tension is maintained on the muscles being stretched.

There are a number of things that can cause injury with this method. Too much tension can be applied to the muscles by the partner, the stretcher can lose concentration and stop contracting the opposite muscle group, or *overzealous athletes can turn something subtle into a contest.* This method is for PNF-trained professionals only.

A trained assistant with good anatomical and neuromuscular knowledge is an absolute necessity for proper PNF stretching. This is the main reason for most athletes to avoid these types of stretches. Fellow athletes, the coach, even the team trainer can not be expected to be fully aware of all the parameters for these functions without extensive education in this specific area of expertise.

PNF STRETCHES

PNF stretches are designed as partner stretches, and if done incorrectly can cause injury (Beaulieu, 1981; Cornelius, 1983).

PNF stretches can be more dangerous than static stretching because more tension is placed on the muscle. With excessive tension on the muscle, the stretch must be monitored closely to reduce the incidence of soft-tissue injury.

PNF techniques have potential benefits, but they also have the potential for damage and negative results. PNF methods can be uncomfortable or even painful, and they require a very motivated person (Moore & Hutton, 1980; Cornelius, 1983).

In addition, experiments have challenged some of the ideas supporting the neurophysiological basis of PNF stretching (Eldred, Hutton, & Smith, 1976; Suzuki & Hutton, 1976).

III. PASSIVE-ACTIVE AND ACTIVE-ASSISTED STRETCHES

Both of these types of so-called stretches employ some "dynamic" movement and some PNF function. They are more difficult and require specifically trained assistance.

In passive stretching the motion or load is performed by an outside agent responsible for the stretch. A partner or special equipment is necessary.

IV. STATIC STRETCHES

Static stretches are accomplished by loading the muscles and allowing the relaxation and sliding elongation described in the *mechanisms of stretching*.

No assistance or special equipment is needed, and the stretches can be done anywhere. This is the type of stretch described in the following chapters for each specific weight-bearing muscle group.

STATIC STRETCHES

Research has demonstrated that permanent length-ening is most favored by *lower force, longer duration stretching* at elevated temperatures (Laban, 1962; Light, Nuzik, Personius, & Barstrom, 1984; Warren, Lehmann, & Koblanski, 1971, 1976).

Static stretching is preferable because it requires less energy expenditure than other methods, it results in less muscle soreness, and it can provide more qualitative relief from muscle soreness (de Vries, 1966, 1980).

It is the best method of stretching for the individual.

The following stretches are the best *primary* stretches for the six weight-bearing muscle groups of the lower extremity. They are the best stretches found that follow all the rules of proper static stretching.

NOTES

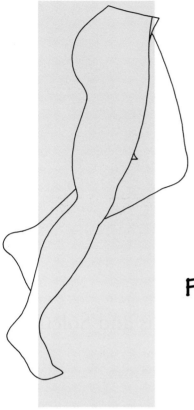

SECTION 3

PRIMARY STRETCHES FOR THE MAJOR WEIGHT-BEARING MUSCLE GROUPS OF THE LOWER EXTREMITIES

In this section the primary stretches for each of the major muscle groups of the lower extremity will be described. If a primary stretch of any muscle group can be done in more than one position, we have included these other positions.

The other stretching positions illustrated and discussed all present problems and can cause injury. Some of the improper stretches illustrated are skill-level stretches, loading more than one major muscle group across the same joint, while placing a heavy load on ligament structures. Others are incorrect because of positioning. The muscles cannot relax back to their resting length if they are contracted, expending energy, in order to maintain that position.

The first two sections of this book explained the structures involved and how they function; this section will help you apply that knowledge to gain the most from your stretches and avoid the long-term damage created by doing them incorrectly.

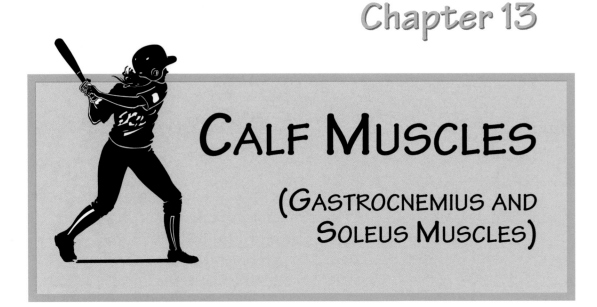

Chapter 13

CALF MUSCLES

(GASTROCNEMIUS AND SOLEUS MUSCLES)

The gastrocnemius and soleus muscles are collectively known as the calf muscles. The gastrocnemius is the more posterior muscle and forms the greater part of the calf.

The soleus is a broad, flat muscle situated immediately underneath (anterior to) the gastrocnemius. The tendons of the gastrocnemius and soleus form the achilles tendon (tendo calcaneus).

The achilles tendon is one of the largest tendons in the body. It is attached to the posterior surface of the heel bone (calcaneus). The tendon is extremely strong and inelastic, but is vulnerable to injury.

We will discuss the two muscles separately. It is important to note that the gastrocnemius muscle crosses both the knee and ankle joint, while the soleus only crosses the ankle joint.

I. GASTROCNEMIUS MUSCLE

A. Anatomy

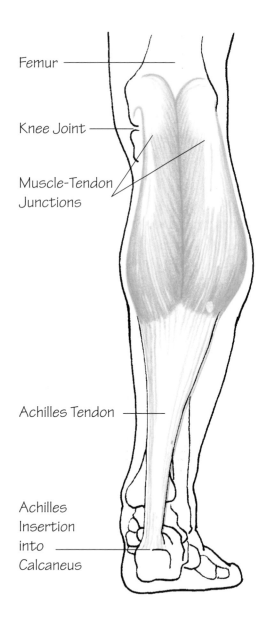

Femur

Knee Joint

Muscle-Tendon Junctions

Achilles Tendon

Achilles Insertion into Calcaneus

The gastrocnemius has two tendons of origin that are attached to the back of the thigh bone (the femoral condyles) above the knee joint. The tendons of origin cross the back of the knee joint, and the muscle-tendon junctions are slightly below the knee joint.

The gastrocnemius has a large, round, fairly short muscle belly whose definition is easily seen in most people. The lower muscle-tendon junction is the starting point of the achilles tendon, which is the tendon of insertion.

The achilles tendon crosses the back (posterior) of the ankle joint and is attached to the heel bone (calcaneus).

B. Biomechanics

The gastrocnemius is one of the most important muscles in the body. When you are walking or running, the *eccentric capacity of the gastrocnemius muscle* determines your *joint position* and *stride length*. To understand how this works, the *eccentric function* of this muscle during the *midstance phase* of the *normal gait cycle* must be understood.

C. Normal Gait Cycle

The normal gait cycle consists of four phases:

1. Swing phase of gait - when the leg is moving through the air.

2. Heel contact - the swing phase of gait ends when the heel contacts the ground. The heel contact phase lasts until the forefoot reaches the ground.

3. Midstance phase of gait - the midstance phase begins when the lateral aspect of the forefoot contacts the ground and lasts until the heel is lifted off the ground. It is during this phase of gait, when the entire foot is on the ground, that *pronation* followed by *resupination* of the foot should occur. Both pronation and resupination are necessary segments of foot motion in the midstance phase of gait for shock absorption and joint repositioning *before* the heel is lifted off the ground.

4. Propulsive phase of gait - this phase lasts from heel lift until the ball of the foot leaves the ground.

II. MIDSTANCE PHASE OF THE NORMAL GAIT CYCLE

A. Pronation

In the midstance phase of gait, the forefoot hits the ground, the leg is moving forward over the foot, and the gastrocnemius is eccentrically contracting. This means the gastrocnemius is elongating, expending energy and doing work: keeping the knee flexed to prevent hyperextension of the knee.

As the foot hits the ground it *pronates* (meaning the arch height decreases and the foot lengthens under the weight-bearing impact). Pronation allows the lower leg muscles, whose tendons cross the ankle joint into the foot, to continue to absorb shock through their elongating *(eccentric)* contractions. *Pronation is a normal and necessary part of every stride.* Pronation allows the joint motion necessary for the lower leg muscles to function fully and absorb shock.

At the end of the pronation phase there is a heavy load on the ligament structures of the pronated foot. The knee is now internally rotated with increased angulation of the patella tendon containing the knee cap, and there is increased stress on the medial knee ligaments. The femur is rotated inward (medially), causing increased load on the hip flexors and external hip rotator muscles, as well as the ligaments of the sacroiliac joints of the pelvis.

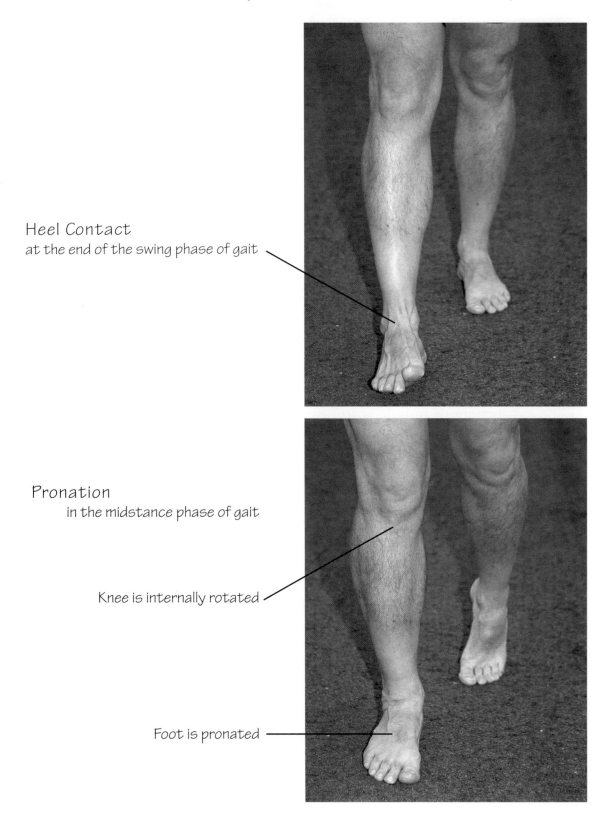

Heel Contact
at the end of the swing phase of gait

Pronation
in the midstance phase of gait

Knee is internally rotated

Foot is pronated

B. Resupination

As the leg continues forward over the foot, which is fixed on the ground, the lower leg muscles start to shorten (concentrically contract) at the end of the pronation phase and lift the bony arch of the foot. This is called *resupination.*

> During resupination, the arch height starts to increase and the foot shortens slightly. The knee externally rotates and realigns the patella mechanism and decreases the load on the medial ligaments of the knee. The femur, hip, and pelvis also attain better alignment. The opposite leg completes the swing phase of gait.

The gastrocnemius muscle is *still eccentrically contracting,* keeping the knee slightly flexed. When the lower leg's forward movement causes the gastrocnemius muscle fibers to slightly exceed their *eccentric capacity,* the overlapping proteins in the myofilaments are extended *past their current resting length.* The muscle spindles react by *myotatic reflex contraction* to stop further elongation of the gastrocnemius to prevent the muscle fibers from being torn.

> This lower motor neuron reflex contraction results in an almost *isometric* contraction of the gastrocnemius muscle. The gastrocnemius is expending energy and resisting further elongation. This isometric contraction of the gastrocnemius muscle lifts the heel off the ground because the leg is continuing forward over the foot, but the gastrocnemius has stopped elongating.

Resupination

Knee externally rotates back to
proper patella mechanism alignment

Swing phase of gait completed on
opposite leg

Arch height increases

Propulsive Phase of Gait

Heel lifts after opposite leg has
completed swing phase

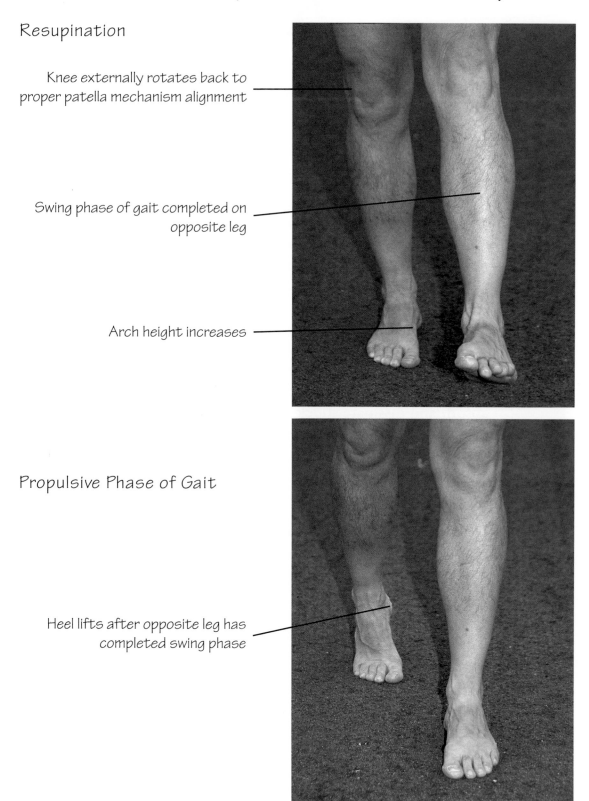

RESUPINATION

This is how the *current resting length* and *eccentric capacity* of the gastrocnemius muscle determines your *joint position* and *stride length*. There must be enough eccentric capacity in the gastrocnemius muscle to allow the lower extremity to complete the full gait cycle.

Pronation followed by resupination are normal segments of the gait cycle. These movements are necessary for proper muscle function and joint motion to absorb and dissipate shock. Proper alignment of the foot, knee, hip, and pelvis is possible *only* if the gait cycle is completed.

III. Structural Damage caused by Shortened Calf Muscles

The calf muscles, especially the gastrocnemius muscle, are always *the first muscles to shorten with repetitive usage and fatigue.* This shortening of the current resting length in the calf muscle reduces the muscle's *eccentric capacity.* This loss of eccentric capacity results in a short stride with poor joint position. Without proper stretches, these muscles will remain shortened for the rest of your life.

A. Stress on the Ligaments of the Lower Extremity

Proper joint position and stride length are not possible with a *shortened gastrocnemius muscle.* The reflex response of the gastrocnemius muscle lifts the heel *prematurely,* while the foot is still pronated. The resupination phase of gait does not occur because of this premature lifting of the heel off the ground by the calf muscles. The pronated foot is not the problem; the calf muscle *lifting the heel while the foot is still pronated* is the problem.

The calf muscles lifting the heel while the foot is still
pronated causes abnormal stress on the ligament structures
of the arch of the foot, especially the large structure known
as the *plantar fascia.*

They also lift the heel while the knee is still internally rotated,
because resupination of the foot and the realignment of the knee
have not occurred. This results in stress to the ligaments of the
knee joint, and excessive pull and angulation of the quadriceps
muscles and tendon (patella tendon) where it attaches to the leg
bone (tibia) below the knee.

Osgood-Schlatter disease,
patella-femoral syndrome,
and chondromalacia are
terms used to describe the
pain and inflammation of
this damage. These medical
terms describe what has
been damaged, *what hurts.*

This excessive stress, with a
resulting accumulation of
microtrauma and secondary
inflammation, is a leading
cause of knee damage in
young athletes; and *in everyone* as we get older.

When a patient has these types of symptoms, the treatment
should focus on the *structural and muscular imbalances* that are
causing the damage. The treatment should be focused on the
cause instead of the symptoms.

Many health professionals are treating
the *symptoms* instead of the cause.

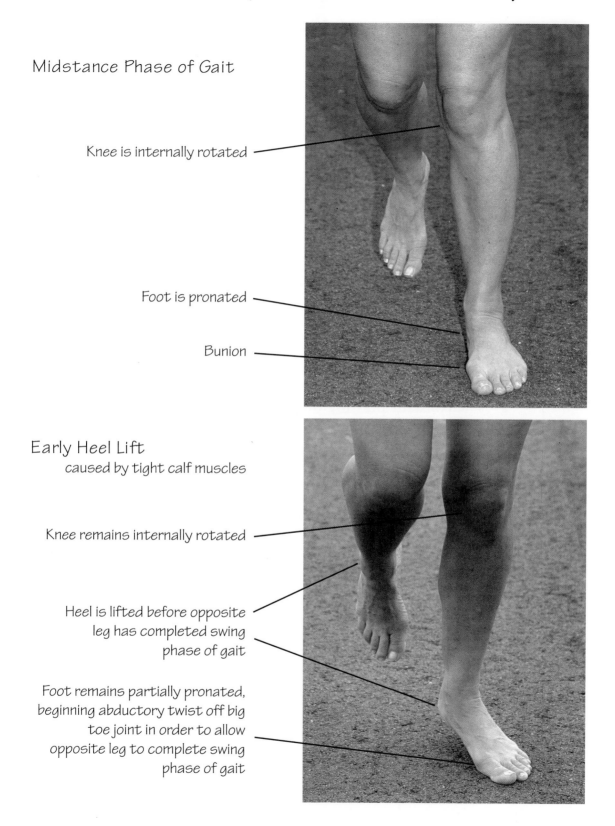

Midstance Phase of Gait

Knee is internally rotated

Foot is pronated

Bunion

Early Heel Lift
caused by tight calf muscles

Knee remains internally rotated

Heel is lifted before opposite leg has completed swing phase of gait

Foot remains partially pronated, beginning abductory twist off big toe joint in order to allow opposite leg to complete swing phase of gait

B. Bunions

All bunions are caused by the short stride and the abductory twist off the big-toe joint (first metatarsal-phalangeal joint) in the propulsive phase of gait which occurs because of the shortened gastrocnemius muscles. When heel lift occurs before you have finished the swing phase of the opposite leg, you spin off the weight-bearing foot in order to gain the time needed to get the opposite leg in front of the pelvis.

- Bunions are a growing bone deformity (bone spur) with ligament stretching and secondary joint dislocation, resulting in degenerative arthritis (osteoarthritis).
  - The constant pressure on the side of the first metatarsal at the joint causes the bone to hypertrophy (the bone continues to enlarge to protect itself), which causes the bone spur (exostosis).
  - The constant stress on the medial ligaments of the big-toe joint (first metatarsal-phalangeal joint) causes microscopic tearing, weakening, and lengthening. This results in the gradual lateral dislocation of the joint.
  - The chronic abnormal loading stress and the resulting inflammation in the joint will lead to destruction of the articular cartilage (osteoarthritis) over a period of time.

- Other factors such as the shape of the big-toe joint, the elasticity of your ligament structures (an inherited characteristic), and the shoes you wear affect how fast a bunion will form. But without the tight calf muscles and the spinning rotation off the side of the big-toe joint in the propulsive phase of gait, no bunion will form.

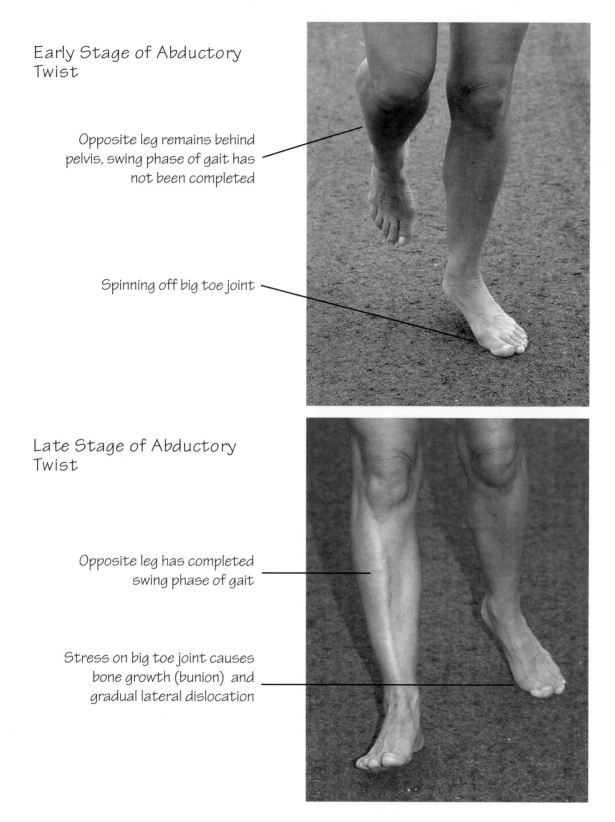

Early Stage of Abductory Twist

Opposite leg remains behind pelvis, swing phase of gait has not been completed

Spinning off big toe joint

Late Stage of Abductory Twist

Opposite leg has completed swing phase of gait

Stress on big toe joint causes bone growth (bunion) and gradual lateral dislocation

BUNIONS

Example:

Walk or run behind your friends and observe which heel lifts the fastest, and how they twist in at the heel as they spin off the inside of their forefoot. The leg with the earliest heel lift and the most abductory twist of the foot will have the larger bunion.

Eliminating the tight calf muscles, by doing proper gastrocnemius muscle stretches, will re-establish good joint position and stride length, and will hinder further development of bunions.

C. Asymmetry

Everyone has a dominant side in terms of muscle coordination and reflex response to loading force. You are either right-handed or left-handed, meaning right or left dominance in neuromuscular control.

The reflex response to loading force is slightly faster on the dominant side. This causes muscles to function slightly quicker, fatigue faster, and shorten more on the dominant side. This results in many people being asymmetrical in their joint position and stride length when walking or running. The resulting muscle imbalances can be seen as asymmetries in movement and even in stance.

ASYMMETRY

Example:

Many people stand with one foot and leg turned out (externally rotated) much more than the other. This asymmetry in their stance results from the gluteal muscles and the external hip rotator muscles of the posterior pelvis being tighter, which externally rotates the femur, turning that leg out more.

For proper
joint position and stride length,
the most important stretch
for everyone
throughout life is the
GASTROCNEMIUS MUSCLE STRETCH.

IV. GASTROCNEMIUS STRETCH: BOTH LEGS AT THE SAME TIME

Isolate the Muscle Group

■ The best position to isolate the gastrocnemius muscles is standing with the entire ball of both feet resting on a raised surface and the heels firmly weight-bearing on the ground. For instance, use a 1-2 inch thick board beneath the ball of your foot.

■ This position enables you to load the gastrocnemius muscles without leaning forward. Leaning forward makes it harder to keep the heels on the ground, which is a *necessity* in a calf-muscle stretch.

■ Hold onto the structure in front of you. For example, stand in front of a door so that you can hold onto the door jam.

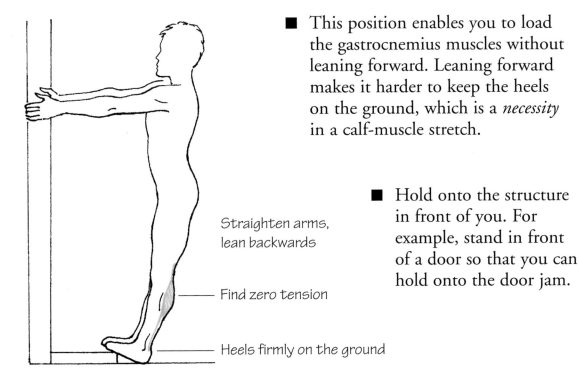

Straighten arms, lean backwards

Find zero tension

Heels firmly on the ground

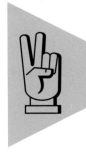

Find Zero Tension

- Standing straight with the forefoot on the raised surface, you will feel tension behind the knee. This is overstretching, because the tension is in the wrong place.
- *Lean backward,* away from the door jam or whatever you are holding onto, to reduce that muscle tension to zero.

- Leaning backward keeps the heels firmly fixed on the ground, the posture remains straight, and the quadricep muscles can relax without the knees buckling. Do not lock the knees by contracting the quadriceps.
- This is the best position for isolating the gastrocnemius muscles in a position where the muscles can relax and slide longer.

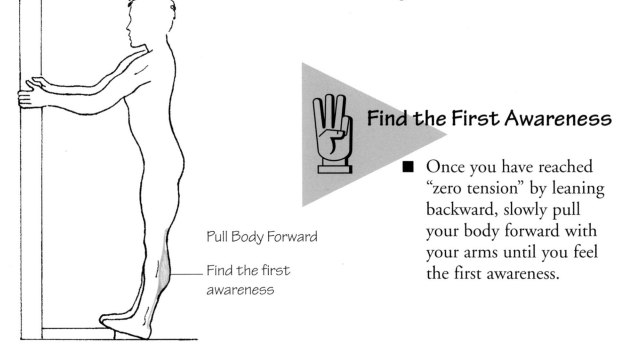

Pull Body Forward

Find the first awareness

Find the First Awareness

- Once you have reached "zero tension" by leaning backward, slowly pull your body forward with your arms until you feel the first awareness.

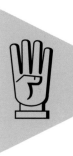

Less is Best

- You have to isolate the first gentle tension, the first awareness, in the middle of the gastrocnemius muscle mass. There should be no sensation of pulling or tension behind the knees.
- The first awareness is subtle! Patience is required until your biofeedback becomes familiar with this gentle tension.

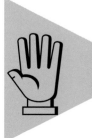

Allow the Loss of Tension

- Hold that position and *allow* that first awareness to diminish and release. When you cannot feel any tension left in the muscle, the sliding elongation (stretch) is completed.

Recommendation:

Repeat the stretch a second time. The only way to gain more length and power is to repeat the process.

A. Advantages of stretching both gastrocnemius muscles at the same time:

There are two reasons for stretching both legs simultaneously. It is the best method of isolating the calf muscles in a proper position where they can relax and elongate, and it also *improves your biofeedback.*

When both legs are loaded at the same time and the first awareness is found, you may feel the tension in only one calf muscle, or one calf muscle slightly more than the other. This is normal. It is the best biofeedback the brain is capable of and the most subtle awareness. The brain is *not registering intensity, it is registering the difference in the two muscles.*

When isolating one calf muscle at a time, people routinely load the calf muscle much harder before the biofeedback registers. At the very least the desired effect is delayed, and damage may result.

The secret is knowing *where to feel that gentle tension,* knowing *where not to feel that tension,* and that less is best. The more gently you load the muscles, the faster they will relax and slide longer.

IV. GASTROCNEMIUS STRETCH: ONE LEG AT A TIME

Sometimes there is nothing convenient on which to place the ball of the feet for the calf stretch, to load both calf muscles at the same time. As an alternative this is how to stretch one leg at a time.

■ To isolate the gastrocnemius muscle, it is important to *keep the heel firmly on the ground.* Position the hips over the heel of the leg being stretched, with the hip and leg forming an angle of about 45 degrees, and keep the back straight. This isolates the gastrocnemius muscle with the heel firmly on the ground.

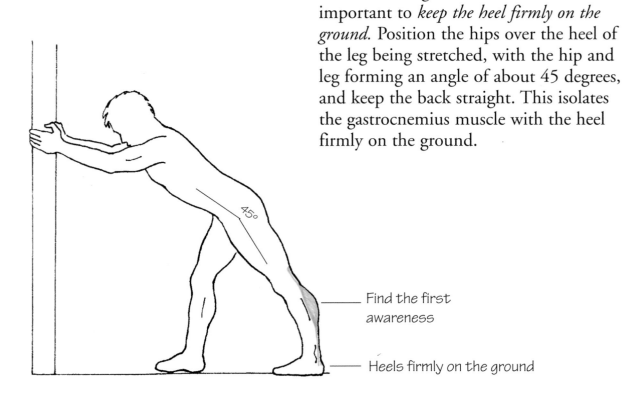

45°

Find the first awareness

Heels firmly on the ground

■ Bend the elbows and the front knee, and lean the whole body as a unit toward the wall. This will increase the tension on the calf muscle, and the hip stays back over the foot to ensure that the heel stays firmly on the ground.

■ If the hip angle straightens it becomes harder to keep the heel on the ground.

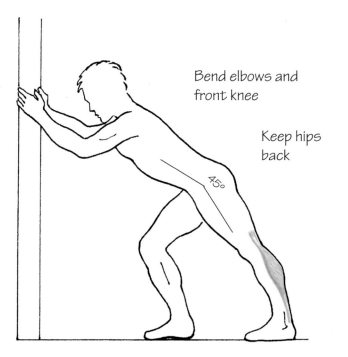

Bend elbows and front knee

Keep hips back

45°

The gastrocnemius muscle cannot relax and slide past its current resting length if it is contracted and expending energy in order to *hold the heel bone in the air.*

V. MISTAKES IN THE GASTROC-NEMIUS MUSCLE STRETCH

A. Overstretching

■ When doing a gastrocnemius muscle stretch you should *never feel any pulling or tension behind the knee.* If you do, you are overstretching. The upper muscle-tendon junctions of the gastrocnemius are slightly below the knee joint and the bulk of the muscle is below the knee.

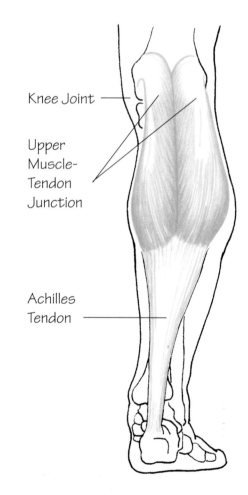

Knee Joint

Upper Muscle-Tendon Junction

Achilles Tendon

■ This overloading of the muscle will delay the relaxation/sliding elonga-tion that is the desired effect; and it may cause tearing and scarring at the upper muscle-tendon junction behind the knee.

■ During the stretch you should never feel any heavy pull in the tendon because it is practically inelastic. NO ONE CAN STRETCH THE ACHILLES TENDON. People who talk about achilles stretches are using old and incorrect terminology. The achilles tendon is a structure composed of very inelastic collagen fiber, and cannot elongate more than 3% without rupture.

Quadriceps contracted

■ The farther you lean forward, as demonstrated in this illustration, the more muscles you have to contract to stabilize this position, and the harder it becomes to keep your heel firmly on the ground.

Heel off the ground

OVERSTRETCHING

The gastrocnemius muscle has demonstrated a myotatic or stretch reflex to stabilize the femur in a standing position to correct an excess shifting of the center of gravity. Some research shows reflex contractions if the angle of the leg over the foot *exceeds forty-five degrees,* even if the heel is on the ground. This is a myotactic response to balance and position, and the gastrocnemius muscle may not relax to the resting length while maintaining this position.

B. Positioning Errors

■ A common mistake is dropping the heels off a step or curb, or leaning forward in a position where the heel comes off the ground. If the heel (calcaneus) is off the ground, the gastrocnemius will remain contracted, expending energy, holding up the bone. This is an isometric contraction by definition. It is *not a stretch*.

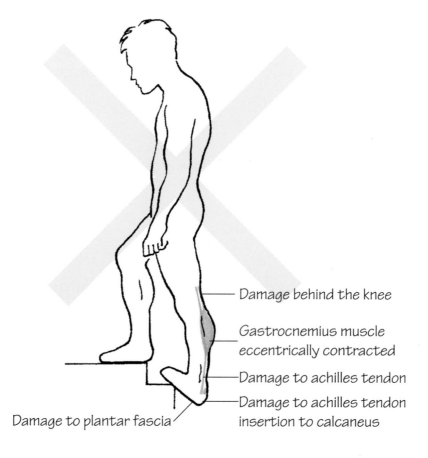

Damage behind the knee

Gastrocnemius muscle eccentrically contracted

Damage to achilles tendon

Damage to achilles tendon insertion to calcaneus

Damage to plantar fascia

■ Because the achilles tendon is stronger than the muscle and the bone, it is the muscle fibers and the periosteum of the heel bone that may be torn. This can lead to chronic tearing and damage to the gastrocnemius muscle, as well as inflammation of the heel (calcaneal periostitis) and achilles tendon (tendonitis).

■ The large tendinous structure of the foot *(the plantar fascia)* is also put under great stress in this position. Even in healthy people this can cause *plantar fasciitis,* a very common and painful problem. In anyone suffering from plantar fasciitis this improper stretch will only make their problem much worse.

■ Some health professionals are prescribing these eccentric drops (the muscles contracted eccentrically to maintain a position) as stretches for treatment of achilles tendonitis and are surprised when their patients' symptoms get worse.

C. Loading Other Structures

■ Other muscles and their tendons are loaded
   when people place their toes against the wall and
   lean into that leg until they feel the calf muscles.

Loads
gastroc-
nemius
muscle

Also loads flexor digitorum longus
and flexor hallucis longus muscles

■ The problem with this position is that it
   creates overloading of the *flexor digitorum longus* and *flexor hallucis longus*
   muscles (shown in the illustration).
   These muscles are part of the deep posterior muscle group against the back of
   the shin bone (tibia). This is a separate
   muscle compartment located underneath
   the gastrocnemius and soleus muscles
   and the achilles tendon.

■ The muscle-tendon junctions of these
   two very important muscles are underneath the achilles tendon, just behind
   the ankle bone (medial malleoli). The
   tendons travel under the medial ankle
   bone and extend all the way to the bottom (plantar aspect) of the toes.

■ The flexor hallucis longus tendon
   is attached to the bottom of the
   big toe (hallux).

■ The flexor digitorum longus tendon divides (bifur-
   cates) into four tendons that attach to the bottom of
   the four smaller toes.

CALF MUSCLES (GASTROCNEMIUS AND SOLEUS MUSCLES)

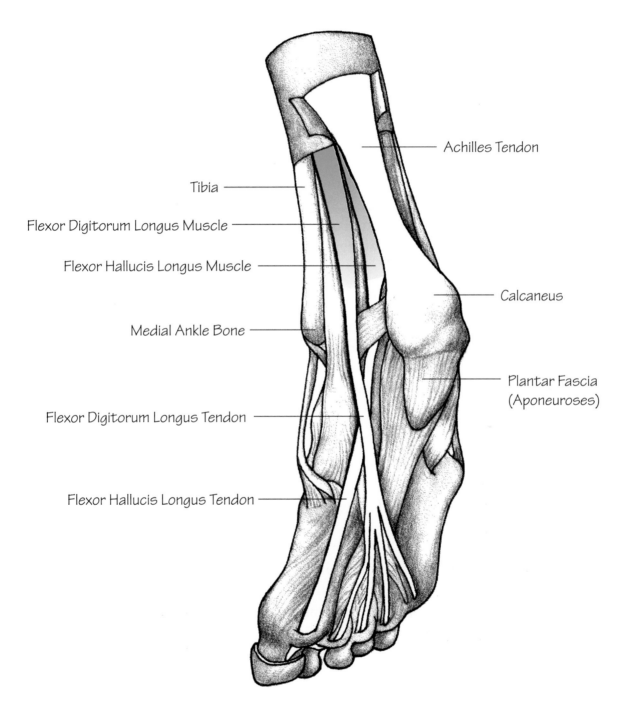

Achilles Tendon

Tibia

Flexor Digitorum Longus Muscle

Flexor Hallucis Longus Muscle

Calcaneus

Medial Ankle Bone

Plantar Fascia
(Aponeuroses)

Flexor Digitorum Longus Tendon

Flexor Hallucis Longus Tendon

■ These muscles are the long flexor muscles of the toes that help stabilize the toes against the ground.

■ When the toes of the foot are extended in the position shown in the illustration, these two small muscles are under a great deal of elongation and tension. If the gastrocnemius muscle is then loaded these small muscles may suffer microscopic tearing and damage.

■ This results in damage at the muscle-tendon junction, tightness and inflammation in the two smaller muscles, and *tenosynovitis* of these muscles' tendons.

TENOSYNOVITIS

Discussion:

Anywhere a tendon is under traction as it is pulled around a bone, such as the inside ankle bone (the medial malleolus), the tendon is surrounded by a tendon sheath.

TENOSYNOVITIS

Tenosynovitis is chronic inflammation of the tendon and the tendon sheath caused by *excessive traction of the tendon* around the bone. The excess traction and microscopic tearing results in the formation of fibrous adhesions of the tendon to the tendon (synovial) sheath. When the muscle is contracted and the tendon moves inside the tendon sheath, these adhesions are broken. This causes a very sharp, quick pain in the area.

Many patients come to my clinic with symptoms of pain around the inside of the ankle and up the back of the shin bone underneath the achilles tendon. They complain of pain on the medial aspect of the ankle *underneath* the achilles tendon, with the soreness extending up the posterior medial aspect of the tibial. They assume that this is an achilles tendon problem.

In reality, this is *tenosynovitis of the long flexor muscle tendons and tendon sheaths* often caused by doing the incorrect stretch described above for months. Prolonged tearing and inflammation to the long flexor muscles can lead to a *posterior compartment syndrome*.

VI. SOLEUS MUSCLE

A. Anatomy

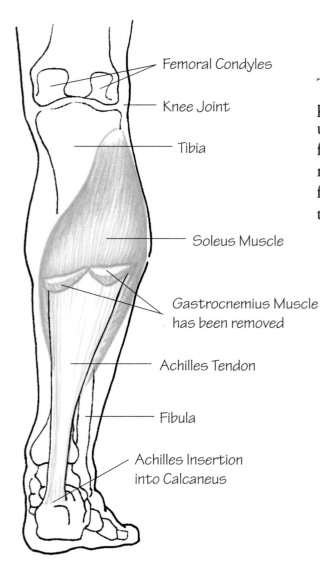

Femoral Condyles

Knee Joint

Tibia

Soleus Muscle

Gastrocnemius Muscle
has been removed

Achilles Tendon

Fibula

Achilles Insertion
into Calcaneus

The soleus originates from the posterior surface of the head and upper third of the shaft of the fibula, the middle third of the medial border of the tibia, and from a fibrous band between the tibia and fibula.

The soleus terminates into a tendon that joins the tendon of the gastrocnemius in forming the achilles tendon.

VII. SOLEUS STRETCH

The soleus muscle shortens with repetitive usage, as does the gastrocnemius muscle. The two muscles work as a unit, with the soleus functioning with the tibia from which it originates.

- The positioning for the soleus stretch is the same as the gastrocnemius stretch, except that in order to isolate the soleus muscle the knee must be flexed enough (15 to 20 degrees) to unload the gastrocnemius muscle completely.

- The heel should be firmly on the ground.

Knee Flexed 15 - 20°

Less than 45° Angle of Ankle

VIII. MISTAKES IN THE SOLEUS MUSCLE STRETCH

A. Positioning Errors

- The soleus is a very active *muscle of posture*. The farther forward the body weight shifts in front of (anterior) the ankle joint, the more the soleus muscle will *involuntarily* contract (myotactic contracture) to stabilize the tibia and fibula.

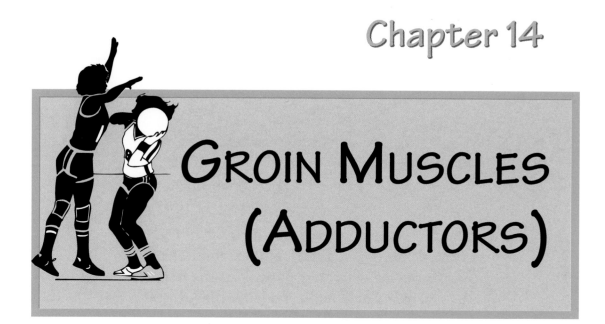

Chapter 14

GROIN MUSCLES (ADDUCTORS)

The groin muscles (the adductors) consist of the five muscles on the inside of the thigh (femur).

The five muscles are:

1. the pectineus

2. the adductor longus

3. the adductor brevis

4. the adductor magnus

5. the gracilis

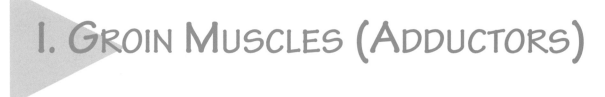

I. GROIN MUSCLES (ADDUCTORS)

A. Anatomy

The groin muscles originate from the bone in the front of the pelvis (pubic rami), and extend down the inside of the leg where they attach to the femur. Only the gracilis muscle tendon crosses the knee joint and attaches to the shin bone (tibia).

B. Biomechanics

These five muscles help stabilize the femur to the pelvis. If these muscles have shortened with repetitive usage and fatigue, they will pull the femur in and the pelvis down in motion, thus increasing knee and back stress.

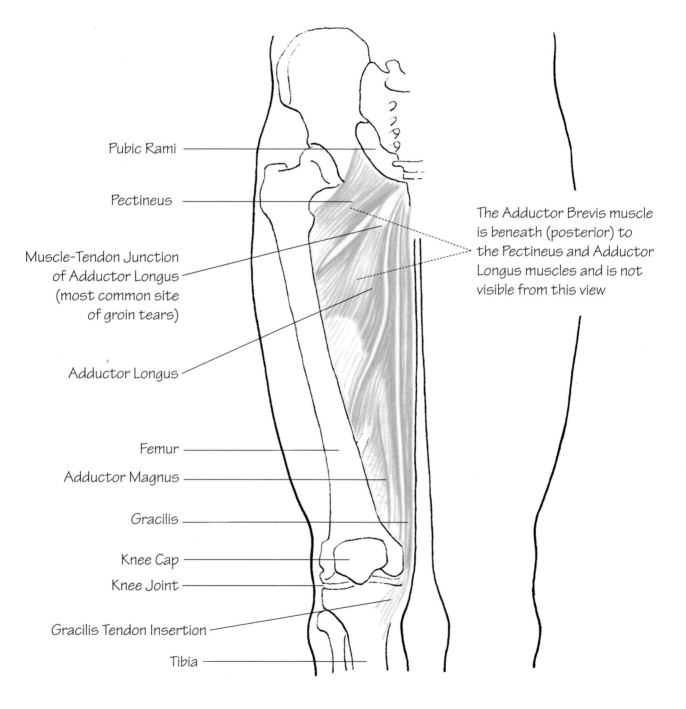

Pubic Rami

Pectineus

Muscle-Tendon Junction
of Adductor Longus
(most common site
of groin tears)

Adductor Longus

The Adductor Brevis muscle
is beneath (posterior) to
the Pectineus and Adductor
Longus muscles and is not
visible from this view

Femur

Adductor Magnus

Gracilis

Knee Cap

Knee Joint

Gracilis Tendon Insertion

Tibia

**Groin Muscles (Adductors)
Anterior View- Right Leg**

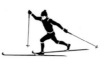

II. SITTING GROIN STRETCH: (SITTING ADDUCTOR STRETCH)

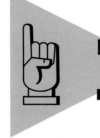

Isolate the Muscle Group

- To isolate the adductors in the best position to allow them to relax and slide past their current resting length, *the stretch must be done sitting.*

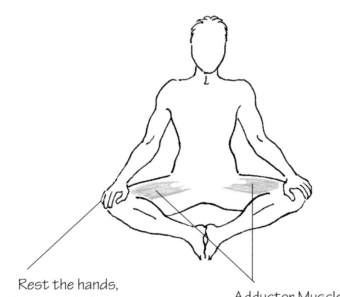

Rest the hands, do not push down

Adductor Muscles

- Rest the back against the wall and place the heels together starting well away from the body. Allow the legs to fall laterally as illustrated. This position isolates the adductor muscles across the hip joint in a position where they are not expending energy to maintain a position.

■ If there is nothing to lean against, use your arms to support the body, and keep the back straight.

Use arms to support body

Keep back straight

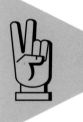

Find Zero Tension

■ Start with the feet and legs far enough from the body so that there is no tension or awareness in the groin muscles.

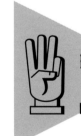

Find the First Awareness

■ Bring the feet toward the pelvis a little at a time until that first gentle tension is felt in the groin muscles.

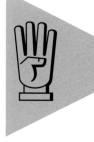

Less is Best

- You may feel only one leg initially. Do not go past that point until the tension is gone.
- Symmetry is everything. The goal is to gain more length in the shorter muscle group and more symmetry with the opposite leg.

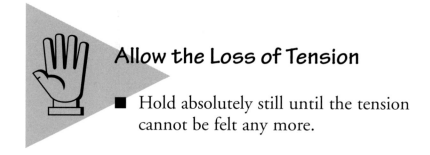

Allow the Loss of Tension

- Hold absolutely still until the tension cannot be felt any more.

III. MISTAKES IN GROIN STRETCHES

A. Overstretching

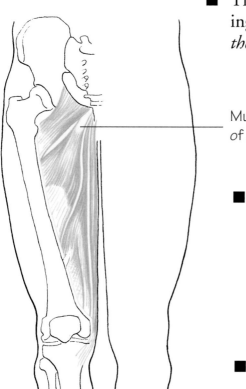

■ The first landmark to learn when stretching the groin muscles *is where not to feel the initial tension.*

Muscle-Tendon Junction
of Adductor Longus

■ The adductor longus has a small, thin tendon of origin arising from the front of the pubic bone. Should the initial tension of the groin stretch be felt in the area of this muscle-tendon junction, it is often an overstretch that will result in tearing and scarring.

■ This tearing of the upper muscle-tendon junction of the adductor longus muscle is the most common *groin tear* injury in sports.

■ If you feel tension in the upper muscle-tendon junction of the adductor longus muscle, reduce the tension by pushing the feet farther away from the body until the tension is felt more in the muscle fibers.

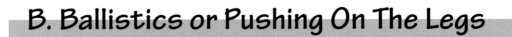
B. Ballistics or Pushing On The Legs

■ *Do not bounce the legs or use your hands to push down on the legs.* Every time the leg is bounced, or you push down on the legs, the muscles contract against the loading force.

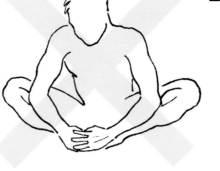

Do not push down on legs with hands or arms

■ This reflex contraction will not allow the muscles to relax back to their current resting length, so the sliding elongation past their resting length cannot happen.

C. Loading Other Structures

(a) Ligaments of the Pelvis

■ The large sacrotuberous ligament that originates from the bone of the pelvis that you sit on (the ischial tuberosity) is one of the main stabilizers of the back of the pelvis.

■ Many adults who bend forward from the pelvis with their legs abducted and externally rotated as illustrated in the groin stretch are causing stress and tearing of the ligament structures of the posterior aspect of their pelvis.

(b) Ligaments of the Spine

- Ligaments of the lower lumbar vertebrae of the spine are also loaded when bending forward in the groin stretch.

- Repeated stress over a long period will weaken these structures.

Ligaments of Lumbar Spine

Ligaments of Posterior Pelvis

Loading Stress on Ligament
Structures of the Pelvis and Lower Spine

Many people get up the morning after exercising and "stretching" and wonder why the back of their pelvis or their lowback feels painful. They do not realize this damage and soreness is the result of the inappropriate positioning while stretching the day before.

D. Positioning Errors

■ NO ONE can stretch their adductors in the standing position illustrated below.

■ The adductors are involuntarily contracted in this position to stabilize the femur to the pelvis against the pull of gravity.

■ This is an involuntary myotactic muscle reflex response to position, balance, and gravity. The adductors cannot be relaxed or the pelvis will fall sideways.

■ If the adductors are voluntarily relaxed, the pelvis will drop and injure the pelvis and/or the femur.

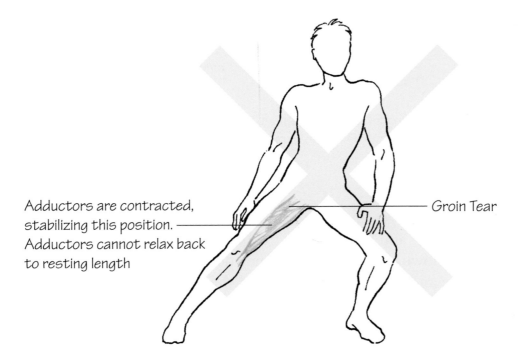

Adductors are contracted, stabilizing this position. Adductors cannot relax back to resting length

Groin Tear

Example:

Many hockey players try to stretch their groin muscles while standing or moving on the ice. Their adductor muscles are contracted to help stabilize the thigh to the pelvis. There can be no sliding elongation of the adductor muscles while standing or moving.

When a bounce or ballistic load is added, this often results in the groin tear they are trying to avoid. This damage will result in increased scar tissue and weakening of the muscle-tendon junctions.

Not only do they gain no benefit from their incorrect stretch, they may actually be causing their groin tears. It is astonishing the number of athletes with groin injuries caused by incorrect groin stretches.

NOTES

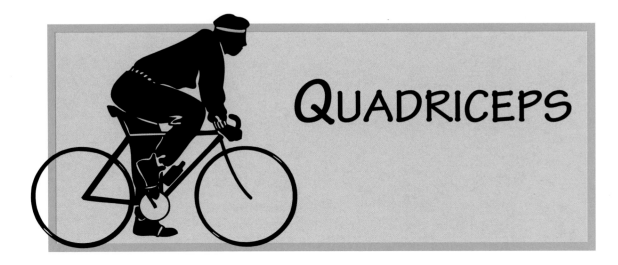

Chapter 15

QUADRICEPS

The four muscles of the front (anterior) of the thigh are the quadriceps.

The four muscles are:

1. the vastus lateralis

2. the vastus intermedius

3. the vastus medialis

4. the rectus femoris

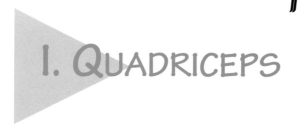

I. QUADRICEPS

A. Anatomy

The Rectus Femoris, the top muscle (anterior) of the quadriceps group, has a tendon of origin from the front of the pelvis. The other three quadriceps have their tendon of origin from the front of the femur.

All of the quadricep muscles' tendons of insertion combine to form the patella tendon.

B. Biomechanics

The quadriceps' main function is to extend (straighten) the leg and stabilize the knee. This muscle group is an important group in terms of power. Sprinters and cyclists need to develop both *strength* and *power* from their quadricep muscles.

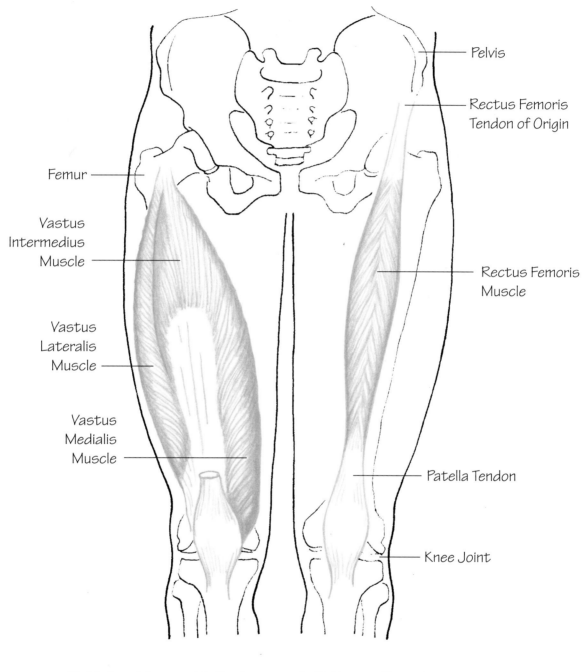

Pelvis

Rectus Femoris
Tendon of Origin

Femur

Vastus
Intermedius
Muscle

Rectus Femoris
Muscle

Vastus
Lateralis
Muscle

Vastus
Medialis
Muscle

Patella Tendon

Knee Joint

**Right Quadriceps with Rectus
Femoris Muscle Removed**

**Left Rectus Femoris
Muscle**

II. QUADRICEPS STRETCH: LYING ON YOUR SIDE

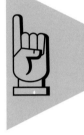

Isolate the Muscle Group

- To isolate the quadriceps, lie on your side as shown in the illustration.
- Flex the knee and hold the *leg* you are stretching just above the ankle; do not hold the foot.

Thigh alignment with Body

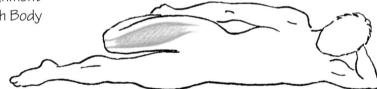

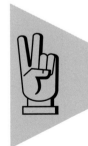

Find Zero Tension

- Start with the thigh far enough in front of the pelvis that there is no awareness of tension in the quadricep muscles.

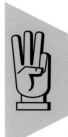

Find the First Awareness

- Find the first gentle tension in the middle of the quadriceps by pulling the leg back with your hand.
- Only a few people with good quadriceps length will need to pull the leg behind the pelvis to find the first awareness.

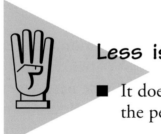

Less is Best

- It does not matter if the leg is still in front of the pelvis when that first tension is found.

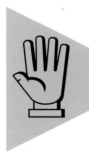

Allow the Loss of Tension

- What does matter is that the position is held long enough for the muscles to relax and elongate. The more this muscle group is elongated the farther back the leg will eventually go.
- Repeat with the other leg.

III. STANDING QUADRICEPS STRETCH

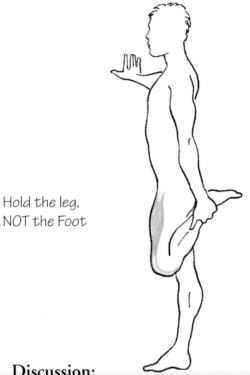

Hold the leg,
NOT the Foot

- The quadriceps stretch can be done standing in the same manner as described when lying on your side.
- In the standing stretch you have weight-bearing stress on other structures, which decreases the subtlety of your awareness in the quadriceps muscles.
- In addition, most people are not patient enough to allow the time necessary for the muscle relaxation/elongation to occur when they are standing.

Discussion:

The *rectus femoris* muscle is longer than the other three quadricep muscles, and its tendon of origin is attached to the pelvis. The three other quadriceps originate from tendons attached to the femur. To increase the load on the rectus femoris in both stretches discussed above, a subtle forward tilt of the pelvis is necessary. The forward rotation of the pelvis increases the length from origin to insertion of the rectus femoris muscle. This is done to ensure you are not just loading the three shorter quadriceps muscles in these stretches.

IV. MISTAKES IN QUADRICEPS STRETCHES

A. Positioning Errors

■ Don't hold your leg with the opposite hand.

　■ When the *right* leg is held with the *left* hand the thigh (femur) is externally rotated. This takes the quadriceps out of their proper functional alignment.

■ This position also loads at least two of the adductor muscles: the pectineus and the adductor longus. This prevents proper positioning and isolation of the muscle group targeted in the stretch.

B. Loading Other Structures

■ When the *foot* is held instead of the *leg above the ankle* while doing a quadriceps stretch, there is a loading force on the long extensor tendons of the toes.

　■ These tendons originate from the anterior muscle group of the lower leg, whose tendons of origin are attached to the *lateral ligament structures of the knee.*

■ This is another example of loading muscle groups unrelated to the muscle group you intended to stretch. This can cause minor strain over a long period of time, resulting in chronic, low-level injury to the lateral structures of the knee where this muscle group originates.

■ At the very least, the loading of other structures interferes with the awareness of the quadriceps in the stretch. The isolation of the muscle group and the bio-feedback will not be as accurate.

Loading foot increases stress on anterior muscles of the leg

C. Injuries

DO NOT put the knee in a weight-bearing position
on the ground for any stretch.

- The knee cap (the patella bone) is part of the
  patella tendon. The posterior surface of the
  patella is covered with articular cartilage. When
  the quadriceps muscles are contracted they extend the knee, using the patella tendon as a
  pulley system across the knee joint.

  - The articular cartilage on the underside
    of the patella, gliding over the articular
    cartilage of the femur, keeps the tendon
    from fraying and breaking down.

- People that must kneel on the knee cap in a
  working situation will often develop damage
  to the articular cartilage of the knee cap and
  the femur (chondromalacia). This is caused by
  constantly driving the two articular surfaces
  against each other with great force. This is an
  unfortunate occupational hazard.

■ It has become popular to kneel down while holding the foot and loading the quadricep muscles as a stretch. *To do this as a stretch is wrong.*

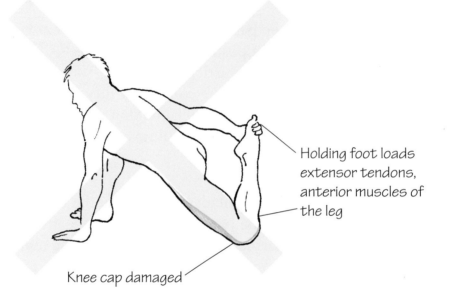

Holding foot loads extensor tendons, anterior muscles of the leg

Knee cap damaged

■ When the quadriceps are loaded with the knee on the ground, traction is applied to the patella tendon that greatly increases the *force of compression* between the knee cap and the femur, causing damage to the articular cartilage of the knee cap and femur.

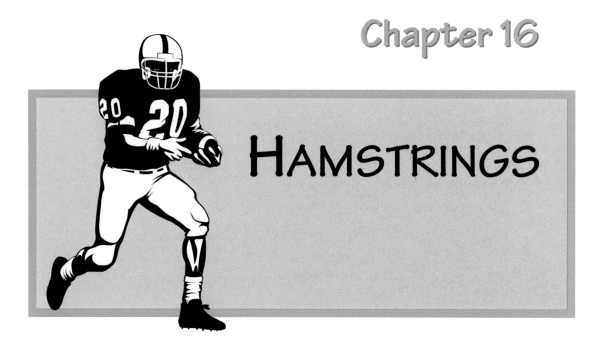

Chapter 16

HAMSTRINGS

The three muscles of the back
of the thigh are the hamstrings.

The three muscles are:

1.   the semitendinosus

2.   the semimembranosus

3.   the biceps femoris

I. HAMSTRINGS

A. Anatomy

All three hamstring muscles have tendons of origin from the bone you sit on (the ischial tuberosity).

The semitendinosus and the semimembranosus are the medial hamstring muscles, which have tendons of insertion crossing the back of the knee on the inside (medial side).

The biceps femoris muscle is the lateral hamstring whose tendon of insertion crosses the back of the knee on the outside (lateral side).

The lower muscle-tendon junctions of the hamstring muscles are approximately 4-8 inches above your knee, depending on the length of your leg.

There is NO hamstring muscle behind the knee!

B. Biomechanics

The hamstrings extend the thigh (femur) on the pelvis and flex the knee. They are very important muscles in terms of acceleration and jumping. They are also very important muscles of position and posture.

The hamstring muscles can only be isolated in a proper stretching position while *sitting or lying on the back.*

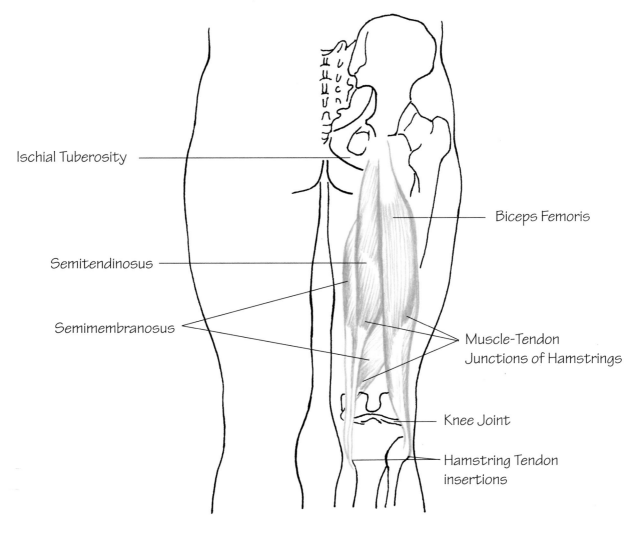

Ischial Tuberosity

Biceps Femoris

Semitendinosus

Semimembranosus

Muscle-Tendon
Junctions of Hamstrings

Knee Joint

Hamstring Tendon
insertions

**Posterior View of
Right Leg**

II. SITTING HAMSTRING STRETCH

☝ Isolate the Muscle Group

■ To isolate the left hamstring muscles in proper sitting position, start with the left leg at a 90° angle to the pelvis.

■ Place the arms on the ground behind the pelvis, and sit with a straight back so that the posterior ligaments of the pelvis and spine are not loaded.

■ Bend (flex) the right knee just enough to allow the right leg to fall sideways as shown.

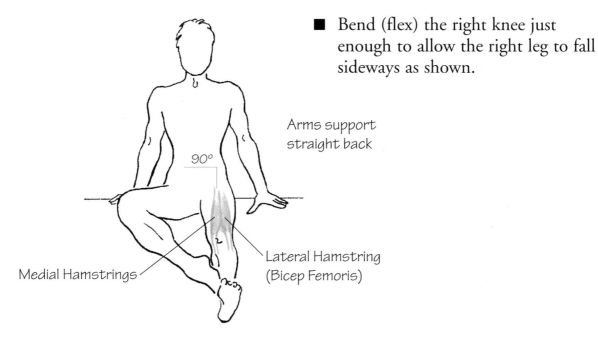

Arms support
straight back

90°

Medial Hamstrings

Lateral Hamstring
(Bicep Femoris)

**Anterior (Frontal) view of hamstring muscles
with femur and all other muscles removed**

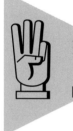

Find Zero Tension

- Move the arms and upper body backward until there is no tension or awareness felt in the hamstrings.

    - Always start where there is no tension or awareness in the hamstrings.

Find the First Awareness

- Move the arms and upper body forward, maintaining a straight back, and find the first awareness in the hamstrings.

    - Often the first awareness will be felt behind the knee where there are no hamstring muscles. There are only *tendons of the hamstring muscles* behind the knee, and other structures such as the *joint capsule* of the knee.

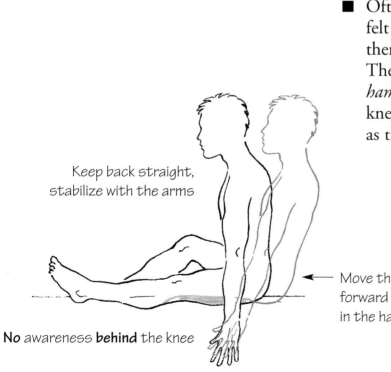

Keep back straight, stabilize with the arms

Move the arms and upper body forward to find the first tension in the hamstring muscles.

No awareness **behind** the knee

■ 139 ■

■ Reduce the tension in very small increments by
moving the arms and upper body backward until
the tension is felt only in the hamstrings muscles
at *least a hand's width above the knee.*

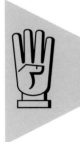

Less is Best

■ The more gentle the initial
muscle load, the faster the
muscle will relax back to its
resting length, and the actual
elongation can begin.

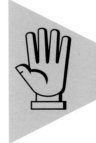

Allow the Loss of Tension

■ The static tension must be held long
enough for the relaxation/sliding
elongation to happen. Remember,
you cannot time stretches.

III. HAMSTRING STRETCHES LYING ON THE BACK

Isolate the Muscle Group

■ Lying on the back to isolate the hamstring muscles is the best way to avoid placing weight-bearing stress on the ligaments of the pelvis and spine.

■ Keep the other knee bent with the foot flat on the floor. This reduces the rotation in the pelvis and negates any load on the hip flexors of the bent leg.

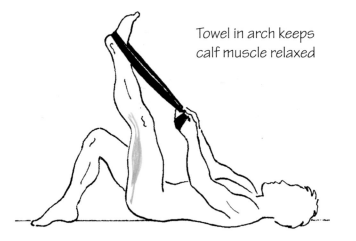

Towel in arch keeps calf muscle relaxed

■ The better the isolation, the fewer structures loaded, the better the biofeedback.

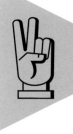

Find Zero Tension

■ The hands can be used to gently support the leg, but it is better isolation to use a towel or a belt to hold the leg as illustrated.

   ■ MAKE SURE that the towel is in the arch of the foot like a stirrup so the forefoot is not loaded, which would cause the calf muscle to tighten.

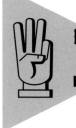

Find the First Awareness

■ Find the first awareness in the hamstring muscles by pulling the leg toward your head. If the first awareness is close to or behind the knee, gradually reduce the tension until the tension moves into the muscle fibers of the hamstrings, at least a hand's width above the knee joint

Less is Best

■ The more gentle the initial muscle load, the faster the muscle will relax back to its resting length.

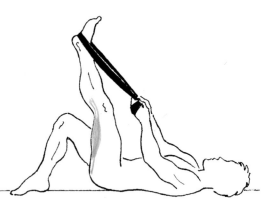

Allow the Loss of Tension

IV. THE WALL STRETCH

People with very tight hamstring muscles can isolate their hamstrings by lying flat on the ground and placing the heels of the feet on a wall. In this position the wall holds the legs, so there is less strain on the arms. The hamstrings can be isolated in a position where they can relax and slide past their resting length in a comfortable position.

■ The tension in the hamstrings is adjusted by two methods in this position.

■ Larger adjustments of the tension on the hamstring muscles are made by sliding the hips closer to the wall to increase the tension, or away from the wall to decrease the tension.

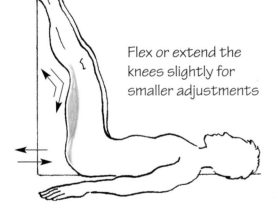

Flex or extend the knees slightly for smaller adjustments

■ Smaller, more subtle adjustments can be made by straightening (extending) the knee for more tension, or bending (flexing) the knee for less tension.

■ Because all three hamstring tendons cross the back of the knee, *all hamstring stretches* should take advantage of the knee movement to adjust the muscle tension.

Move hips closer or farther from the wall for larger adjustments

■ The rules of where and where not to feel the tension do not change, regardless of which proper position you choose as a stretch. Remember, do not feel any tension behind the knee, because there is no hamstring muscle behind the knee.

V. ISOLATING THE MEDIAL OR LATERAL HAMSTRINGS

The medial or lateral hamstring muscles can be isolated in any of the proper stretches discussed here. This not only allows you to concentrate on a specific hamstring muscle when it has a problem, it gives you the ability to test your hamstrings and identify an imbalance before a serious problem occurs.

Isolate Medial Hamstrings

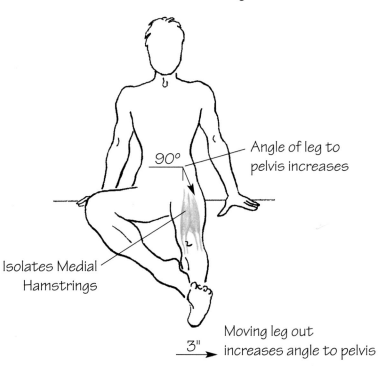

90°

Angle of leg to pelvis increases

Isolates Medial Hamstrings

3"

Moving leg out increases angle to pelvis

Anterior (Frontal) view of hamstring muscles

■ To isolate the medial hamstrings, move the leg out about three inches, widening the angle of the leg to the pelvis. This increases the length of origin to insertion of the medial hamstring muscles (semimembranosus and semitendinosus muscles). Most people can do this with no change in muscle tension, or the tension moves slightly to the inside (medially) of the hamstrings.

■ To isolate the lateral hamstring, move the leg in about three inches, decreasing the angle of the leg to the pelvis. This increases the length of origin to insertion of the lateral hamstring muscle (biceps femoris). Most people will feel more tension and feel the tension move toward the back of the knee because the lateral hamstring is often tighter than the medial hamstrings.

■ Continue isolating the lateral hamstring and reduce the tension in the muscle until the tension is felt only in the muscle fibers well above the knee.

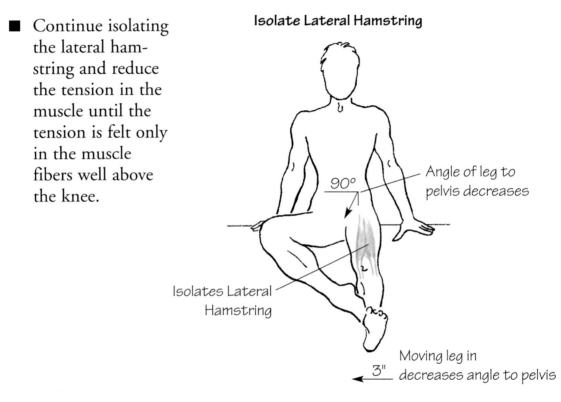

Isolate Lateral Hamstring

90°

Angle of leg to pelvis decreases

Isolates Lateral Hamstring

Moving leg in decreases angle to pelvis

3"

Anterior (Frontal) view of hamstring muscles

The reason most people feel a greater tension when they move the leg medially to isolate the lateral hamstring is because the traditional stretch often taught is incorrect, and places more tension on the medial hamstrings.

VI. MISTAKES IN HAMSTRING STRETCHES

A. Positioning Errors

■ As described previously, increasing the angle of the leg to the pelvis during a hamstring stretch isolates the medial hamstrings. Spreading the legs increases the length of origin to insertion and places more tension on the medial hamstrings (semitendinosus and semimembranosus muscles). The length of origin to insertion and the tension on the lateral hamstring is *decreased*.

■ Just as spreading the legs increases the angle of the leg to the pelvis, pulling the other leg up toward the pelvis increases the angle of the pelvis to the leg that is being stretched. Both of these are training errors and should be avoided.

■ In the position illustrated, the medial hamstrings of the right leg are placed under more tension. This is the reason so many athletes have tight lateral hamstrings.

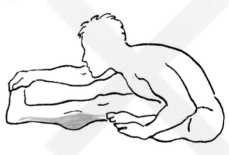

Pulling the left leg this far toward the pelvis rotates the pelvis away from the right leg

■ In the sitting stretch, start with the opposite leg flexed and out of the way, but keep the pelvis at 90° or less to the leg that you are stretching as described on page 136.

B. Loading Other Structures

1. The sitting stretch can damage the posterior ligaments of the lumbar spine and the pelvis if you lean too far forward in this position. Leaning forward increases the loading stress on these ligaments, resulting in insidious tearing and scarring of these structures.

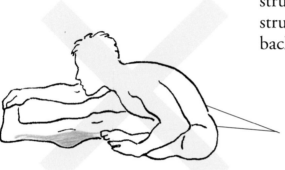

Even if no damage is caused to these structures, the loading of the ligament structures interferes with the biofeedback from the hamstrings.

Loads ligaments of posterior pelvis and lumbar spine

2. Never do a hamstring stretch with the opposite knee weight-bearing on the ground in the position illustrated below. This causes tearing, scarring, and weakening of the medial ligaments of the knee joint.

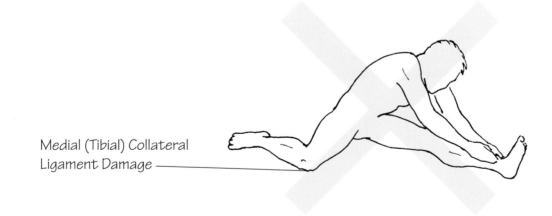

Medial (Tibial) Collateral Ligament Damage

3. Never grab the toes in a hamstring stretch. The gastrocnemius muscle tendons of origin begin above the knee, and the hamstring tendons of insertion all attach to the tibia below the knee. When the calf muscles are placed under loading force simultaneously with the hamstring muscles, the structure often mistakenly loaded and damaged is the posterior joint capsule of the knee.

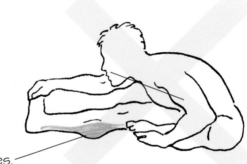

Never grab the toes,
this loads the calf muscles

In this position, ask anyone where they feel "the stretch"; and they always point to BEHIND THE KNEE. There is no hamstring *muscle* behind the knee.

Never load two muscle groups across the same joint at the same time in a *primary stretch*.

C. Incorrect Positioning Due to Involuntary Muscle Contraction

(a) All Standing Hamstring Stretches

There are many examples of improper hamstring stretches. A close look at what the hamstrings do involuntarily in reflex response to standing and bending forward will explain why all standing hamstring stretches are not only wrong, but damage other structures.

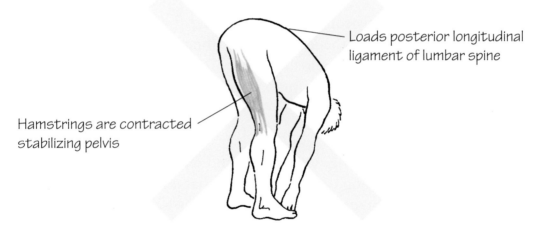

Hamstrings are contracted stabilizing pelvis

Loads posterior longitudinal ligament of lumbar spine

FACT: When a person is standing and bends forward from the pelvis, the hamstring muscles involuntarily contract (myotactic reflex) to stabilize the pelvis against gravity. The hamstrings will remain contracted, stabilizing the pelvis, as long as the person remains bent forward from the hips.

The hamstrings cannot be stretched in any standing position, because they are contracted and expending energy to stabilize the pelvis against the pull of gravity.

When the hamstrings have contracted to their longest eccentric length (eccentric capacity), the pelvis stops rotating forward.

If the person continues to bend forward, they do so by rounding the lower back as they reach for the ground. This transfers loading force into the posterior longitudinal ligament of the lumbar spine.

This will cause tearing, weakening, and lengthening of the posterior longitudinal ligament that stabilizes the spinal vertebrae and spinal disk. As this ligament weakens over a period of years, the instability can lead to hypermobility of the spine and secondary damage, such as a *herniated disk*.

The damage to these ligament structures is insidious, cumulative, and permanent. The resulting spine and sciatic nerve problems may not become symptomatic until years after the initial damage began.

(b) Ballet Bar Stretches

The ballet bar stretch, where one leg is
resting on a chair or a bar or a bench, is also
a very damaging position. Again the damage
is slow, insidious, and permanent.

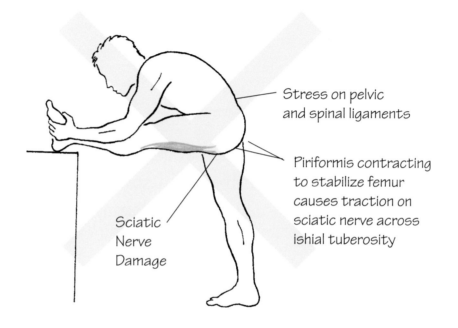

Stress on pelvic
and spinal ligaments

Piriformis contracting
to stabilize femur
causes traction on
sciatic nerve across
ishial tuberosity

Sciatic
Nerve
Damage

Both legs are weight-bearing in this position and the person is bending forward from the pelvis. There is good
evidence that this also causes a reflex contraction of the
hamstring group of both legs to stabilize the pelvis.

In addition, because the femur has rotated on the pelvis and is weight-bearing, the external hip rotators, including the piriformis muscle, are contracted to stabilize the femur. The piriformis muscle anchors the sciatic nerve roots in the posterior hip, especially S2 and S3, and the sciatic nerve plexus is pulled across the bone you sit on (the ischial tuberosity). *See pages 156-158.*

This is called the piriformis syndrome in some studies of sciatic nerve damage.

This repetitive traction of the sciatic nerve is one of the causes of sciatic nerve damage (sciatica or neuropraxic stretching injury). Many young athletes initiate this damage at age eight or nine, but do not become symptomatic until they are much older.

Chapter 17

POSTERIOR HIP MUSCLES

(GLUTEUS MAXIMUS & THE EXTERNAL HIP ROTATORS)

The posterior muscles of the hip are the gluteal muscles and the external hip rotator muscles of the femur.

The gluteal muscles are the gluteus maximus, gluteus medius, and the gluteus minimus.

The external hip rotator muscles are the piriformis, the obturator internus, the obturator externus, the gemellus superior, the gemellus inferior, and the quadratus femoris.

I. GLUTEUS MAXIMUS MUSCLE

A. Anatomy

The gluteus maximus is the largest and most prominent muscle of the back of the hip. It has its tendon of origin attached to many structures of the posterior pelvis. Most of its tendon of insertion is attached to the iliotibial tract (I.T. Band).

B. Biomechanics

The gluteus maximus is the major muscle of the iliotibial band. The iliotibial band stabilizes the knee from the lateral side, and is the largest tendinous structure of the body.

Muscles of the Iliotibial Band

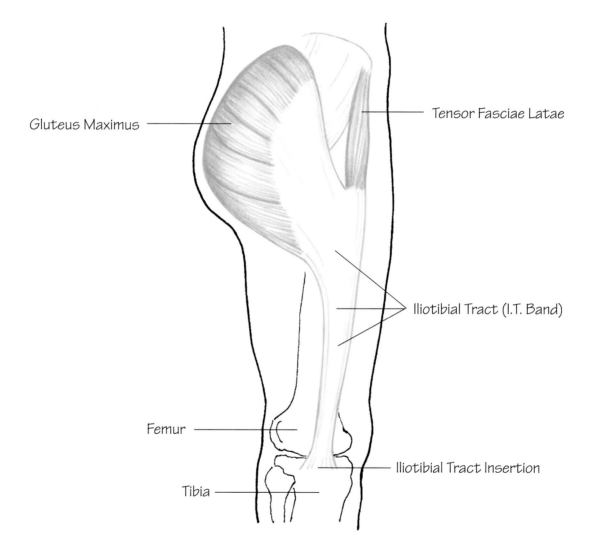

Gluteus Maximus

Tensor Fasciae Latae

Iliotibial Tract (I.T. Band)

Femur

Iliotibial Tract Insertion

Tibia

Lateral View of Right Leg

II. EXTERNAL HIP ROTATOR MUSCLES

A. Anatomy

The six smaller muscles beneath the gluteal muscles are the external hip rotators. These small muscles originate from the tail-bone area (the sacrum), cross the back of the pelvis and the sacroiliac joint, and have tendons of insertion attaching to the posterior aspect of the hip bone (the greater trochanter of the femur).

B. Biomechanics

These are the muscles that stabilize the top of the femur in motion, and which turn the femur externally on the pelvis. Some of these smaller muscles cannot be seen from the posterior view in the illustration. They are beneath (anterior) to the more posterior muscles shown.

The most important of the external hip rotators in terms of injury is the piriformis muscle. The origin of the piriformis muscle is on the anterior surface of the sacrum in the intrapelvic cavity.

External Hip Rotators

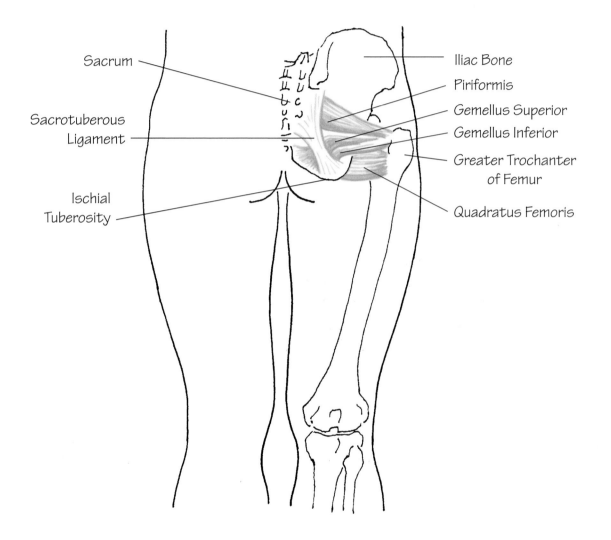

Sacrum

Sacrotuberous
Ligament

Ischial
Tuberosity

Iliac Bone
Piriformis
Gemellus Superior
Gemellus Inferior
Greater Trochanter
of Femur
Quadratus Femoris

Posterior View of Right Leg

III. RELATIONSHIP OF THE POSTERIOR HIP MUSCLES AND THE SCIATIC NERVE ROOTS

Two of the five sciatic nerve roots which form the sciatic nerve plexus, S2 and S3, often pass through the origin of the piriformis muscle (Grant's Atlas, 1972).

The sciatic nerve relationship with the piriformis muscle varies from person to person. In some cases, one or both parts of the sciatic nerve can perforate the piriformis, while in others it passes above or below the muscle; it may even split and pass around the muscle (Janse, 1976; Kendall, Kendall, & Boynton, 1952; Lewin, 1944).

The sciatic nerve roots S2 and S3 have branches separating after passing through the piriformis muscle to become the pudendal nerves to the pelvic cavity. The piriformis muscle cannot be in spasm or excessive tightness for a prolonged period without causing traction on the sciatic and pudendal nerves, resulting in secondary nerve dysfunction.

Long-term symptoms of sciatic nerve damage (sciatica) include everything from numbness and weakness to pain and muscle spasms, especially in the muscles of the posterior hip and down the back of the leg, depending on what portion of the nerve roots are damaged

Origin of Piriformis Muscle, Sciatic Nerve Roots

Lumbar Spine — L3

L4

L5 — Sacrum

S1

Sciatic Nerve Roots L4, L5, S1

S2 — Iliac

Sciatic Nerve Roots S2 and S3

S3

Sciatic Nerve

S4

Piriformis Muscle

S5

Pudendal Nerve

Coccyx (Tailbone)

Coccygeus Muscle

Anterior View of Sacrum

Damage to the pudendal nerve can cause *loss of bladder control, bowel functions, even sexual dysfunction.* It is not uncommon to see patients that have had increasing sciatic nerve problems and hip pain also complaining of periodic episodes of incontinence.

NERVE DAMAGE

Interference with reproductive function has been indicated. This is attributed to damage to the pudendal nerves and blood vessels (Retzlaff et al., 1974).

Because of the interrelationship of the posterior hip muscles, especially the piriformis muscle and the sciatic nerve roots, this stretch is of great importance to anyone that has lowback problems, sacroiliac joint and pelvic pain, and of course sciatic nerve problems.

It is sadly overlooked or done incorrectly in many treatment therapies.

IV. GLUTEUS MAXIMUS AND EXTERNAL HIP ROTATOR STRETCH

Isolate the Muscle Group

■ The best position to isolate the gluteus maximus and the external hip rotators of the right hip is lying flat on the back. Keep the left foot flat on the ground with the knee bent (flexed). Cross the right leg as illustrated.

■ This position isolates the large muscle of the iliotibial band (gluteus maximus) and the six smaller muscles crossing the back of the pelvis (external hip rotators) to attach to the back of the hip bone (greater trochanter of the femur).

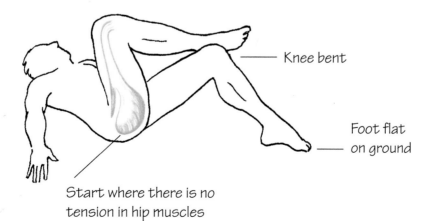

Knee bent

Foot flat on ground

Start where there is no tension in hip muscles

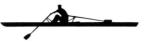

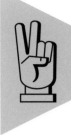

Find Zero Tension

- If you feel tension in the posterior hip muscles of the right leg, gradually move the left foot farther away from your body until there is no tension.

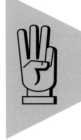

Find the First Awareness

- Gradually bring the left foot toward the buttocks until you feel the first awareness of tension in the posterior muscles of the right hip.

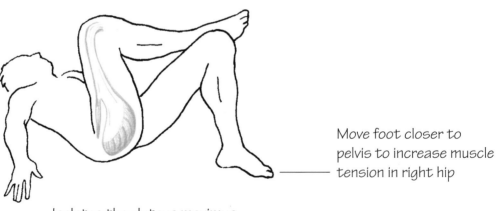

Move foot closer to pelvis to increase muscle tension in right hip

Isolates the gluteus maximus and external hip rotators

- If the first awareness has not been found when the left foot is as close to the body as possible, *only* then would you lift the left leg off the ground until you find the first awareness of tension in the right hip muscles.

■ Use your hands to lift the leg, grasping the thigh just beneath the knee. If you find that you must lift your upper back and head off the ground to reach the thigh, you can use a towel behind the thigh. Pull on the towel with your hands to lift the leg.

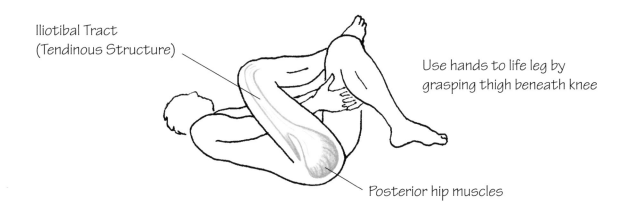

Iliotibal Tract (Tendinous Structure)

Use hands to life leg by grasping thigh beneath knee

Posterior hip muscles

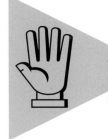

Less is Best

■ Do not go past that position until that first gentle awareness is gone.

Allow the Loss of Tension

■ Remember, pulling harder only delays the muscle relaxation and places more traction on the sciatic nerve roots S2 and S3.

V. MISTAKES IN POSTERIOR HIP MUSCLE STRETCHES

A. Overstretching

Referring to the illustrations of these structures it is evident that you should not feel anything down the outside of the leg of the posterior hip muscles you want to stretch. There is no muscle in the iliotibial band. It is an inelastic collagen structure, really a large tendon. If you feel a tension down the outside of the leg, you are overstretching and may cause microscopic tearing.

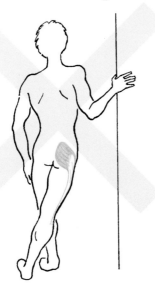

Posterior hip muscles are contracted to stabilize position

B. Positioning Errors

Many people are taught to lean into the wall with their hips rotated sideways as illustrated. *This is not a stretch.* When leaning sideways in a standing position, the muscles of the iliotibial band contract to stabilize the knee from the lateral side. The external hip rotators contract to stabilize the femur in this position.

Once again, this a position where these muscles are contracted in response to gravity and balance. They cannot relax because they are stabilizing this weight-bearing position. This position can cause tearing of the iliotibial band insertion in the lateral aspect of the tibia and also pain in the hip from the friction of the hip bone (greater trochanter) underneath the iliotibial band.

C. Loading Other Structures

Sitting and pulling the hips sideways is often a problem, especially if the ischial tuberosity (the bone you are sitting on) is lifted off the ground. This will cause traction of the sciatic nerve underneath the ischial tuberosity.

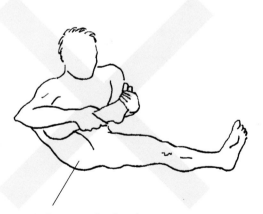

Lifting ischial tuberosity, traction on sciatic nerve

Sitting and twisting the pelvis and spine in one direction while pulling the left leg across the pelvis causes the external hip rotators to contract. This places traction on the proximal nerve roots of the sciatic nerve.

The sciatic nerve trunk passes beneath the bone you are sitting on (the ischial tuberosity). With the proximal nerve roots under traction, especially S2 and S3 which often pass through the piriformis muscle, and the nerve trunk being pulled under the ischial tuberosity, this position can cause sciatic nerve damage.

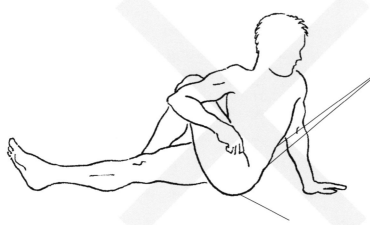

Weight-bearing load and rotational stress on ligament structures of pelvis and spine

Sciatic nerve damage

In the sitting position there is also unnecessary weight-bearing stress and rotation on the *ligaments* of the pelvis and spine. This is *unnecessary in order to stretch this muscle group,* and may cause damage.

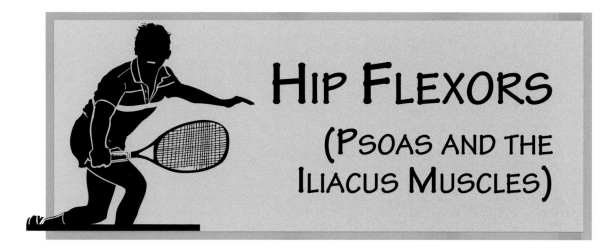

Chapter 18

HIP FLEXORS
(PSOAS AND THE ILIACUS MUSCLES)

The hip flexors are comprised of two muscles, the psoas and the iliacus. Together these two muscles form one of the strongest muscle groups in the body.

I. PSOAS AND ILIACUS MUSCLES

A. Anatomy

(a) Psoas Muscle

The psoas is a very long muscle whose tendons of origin are anchored to the anterior/lateral portion of the entire lower spine. These tendons originate on the anterior surface of the transverse processes, the lateral borders of the vertebral bodies, and the corresponding *intervertebral disks* of the spine from *T12* through *L5*.

The psoas separates from the spine at the 5th lumbar vertebrae and transverses through the pelvic girdle, passes under the inguinal ligament in front of the capsule of the hip joint, and its tendon of insertion attaches to the inside of the thigh bone (the lesser trochanter of the femur).

Psoas and Iliacus Muscles

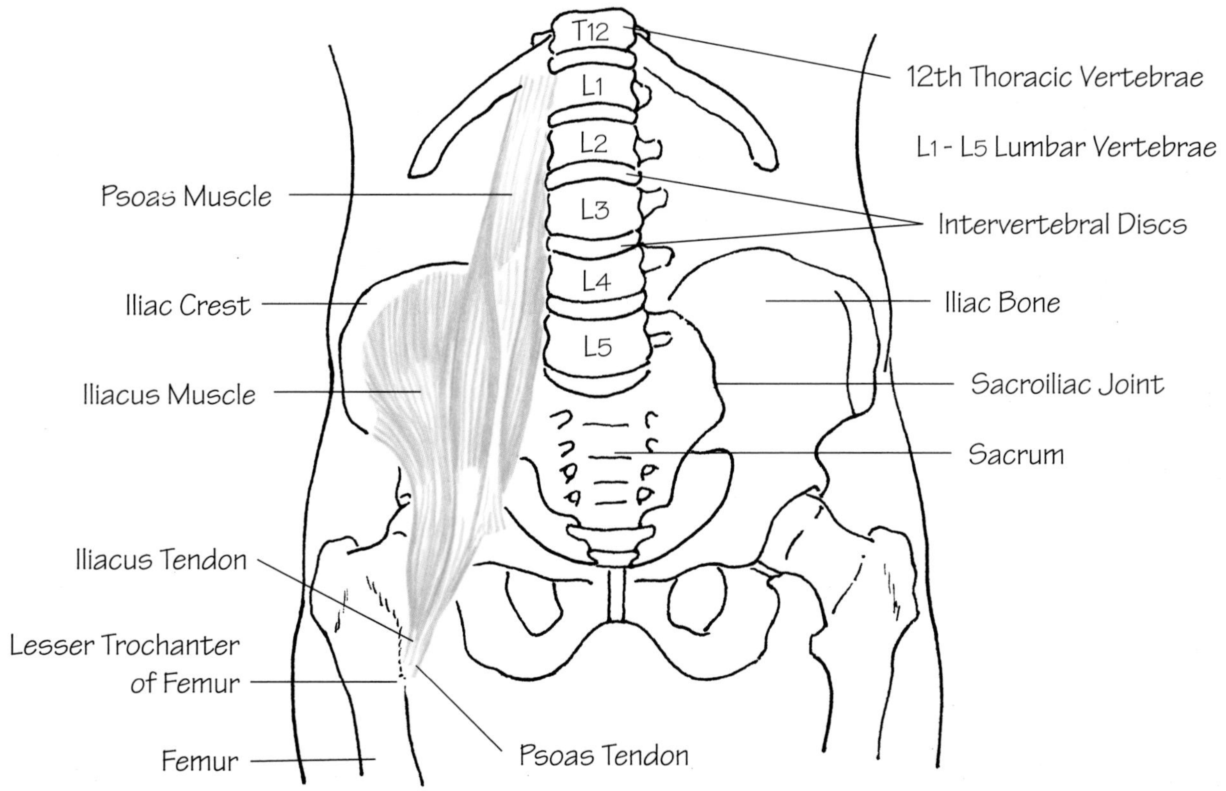
T12
L1
L2
L3
L4
L5
12th Thoracic Vertebrae
L1 - L5 Lumbar Vertebrae
Psoas Muscle
Intervertebral Discs
Iliac Crest
Iliac Bone
Iliacus Muscle
Sacroiliac Joint
Sacrum
Iliacus Tendon
Lesser Trochanter of Femur
Femur
Psoas Tendon

Anterior View of the Lower Spine, Pelvic Girdle and Femurs

(b) Iliacus Muscle

The iliacus muscle originates from tendons that are anchored to the inside of the pelvis, with tendinous slips coming off many of the structures that hold the posterior/lateral aspect of the pelvis together. These tendons originate from the upper two-thirds of the iliac fossa, the internal border of the iliac crest, the anterior sacroiliac, lumbosacral and iliolumbar ligaments, and the ala of the sacrum.

The iliacus also passes beneath the inguinal ligament, where most of its tendon of insertion converges into the lateral/dorsal side of the tendon of the psoas, with the tendon of insertion ultimately inserting into the inside of the lesser trochanter of the femur.

B. Biomechanics

The iliopsoas complex (hip flexors) are the muscle group that is the prime mover when you lift the thigh to the trunk, and when you bend the trunk to the thigh, *as in sitting up from a prone position.*

This is why full sit-ups, especially fixed-leg sit-ups, are not a good abdominal exercise. The hip flexors are the prime movers in this exercise, and have the mechanical advantage necessary to lift the trunk toward the legs.

The farther in front of the axis of the hip joint the upper body is, and the more extended the femur is behind the axis of the hip joint, *the more postural contraction in the hip flexors.*

The hip flexors play an important role in postural balance, and are active in the relaxed standing position (Basmajian, 1978; Greenlaw, 1973; Shy Yan Ng, 1978).

This is precisely why the "runner's stretch" illustrated here is another example of a dynamic contraction, not a stretch. In this position the hip flexors are contracted, doing work, and expending energy in order to stabilize the trunk on the lower extremity.

Runner's "Stretch"

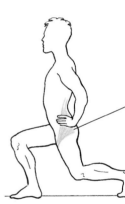

Hip flexors contracted to stabilize femur to pelvis and spine

A Good Mobilization Exercise

Taking the muscles of a muscle group to their longest length of contraction is a good mobilization exercise, and will keep the sarcomeres at the ends of the muscles functioning. As discussed in the segment on dynamic "stretches," one can even increase the amount of sarcomeres at the ends of the muscle in this fashion.

II. HIP FLEXOR STRETCH

A. Stretching Alone

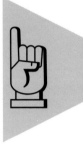

Isolate the Muscle Group

- To isolate the hip flexors (the iliopsoas complex), in a position where they can relax and slide past their resting length, lay flat on your back (supine) on a table.

- In this position the femur is allowed to abduct and drop, placing a mild tension on the iliopsoas complex.

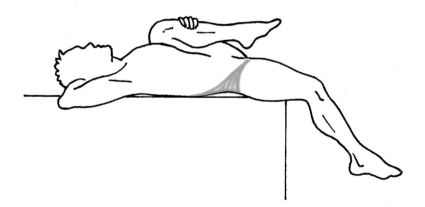

■ It is vital that the lumbar spine remain flat on the table. If the lowback arches off the table, the pull of the psoas muscle on the vertebrae and the intervertebral disk is increased. This may cause injury to the intervertebral disk.

■ Having the opposite leg held firmly to the chest while doing this stretch helps keep the lowback flat on the table.

■ In this position it is hard to isolate the hip flexors because the hanging leg loads other muscle groups. The sartorius and gracilis muscles are loaded, and to a lesser degree the quadriceps muscles.

■ Although this is the only position I am aware of to isolate the hip flexors, I remain unconvinced that anyone can truly isolate the hip flexors enough to benefit from this stretch when doing it alone.

B. Stretching with a Partner

■ With a partner assisting you, the lower leg is held with the knee slightly flexed. With the lower leg supported, the other muscle groups can be minimized or eliminated, and you gain better isolation of the hip flexors.

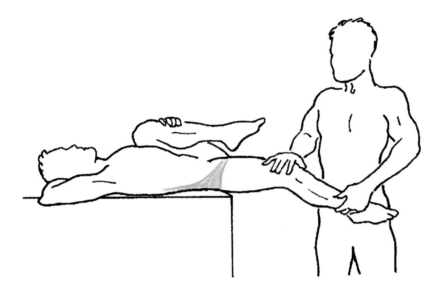

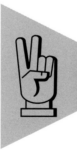

Find Zero Tension

■ The partner supports the lower leg by holding the leg at the ankle, keeping the knee slightly bent. This stops the loading of the sartorius, gracilis, and rectus femoris muscles. As always, start where there is no awareness of tension in the hip flexors.

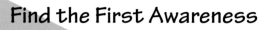

Find the First Awareness

■ The partner can then place a light load on the hip flexors by pushing down and out gently on the thigh with the other hand.

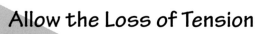

Less is Best

■ Never load these muscles past the first awareness!

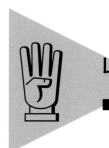

Allow the Loss of Tension

■ The partner must maintain a gentle, steady pressure on the hip flexors and allow these muscles to relax and slide past their current resting length.

CAUTION-CAUTION-CAUTION

This is a difficult stretch, and can cause a great deal of harm if done incorrectly. We advise people not to attempt it without professional help.

NOTES

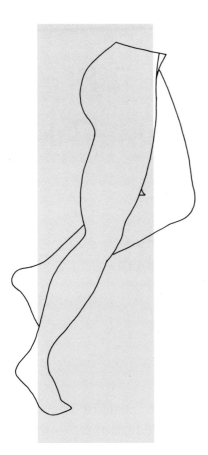

SECTION 4

Easy Reference to Correct Stretches

This section is a quick-reference guide for the reader. Included are the five most practical primary stretches of the weight-bearing muscle groups of the lower extremity for everyone.

As stated previously, a primary stretch is the best stretching position to isolate one muscle group across one joint in a position where that muscle group can relax and slide past their current resting length. This position does not place a significant load on other structures such as the ligaments of joints or the sciatic nerve.

Several of these major muscle groups have more than one proper stretching position. The hamstrings for example, can be stretched sitting or lying on your back. For these muscle groups the stretching position that is the most useful for all ages and for people with extremely tight muscle groups has been chosen.

Anyone that has questions about other stretching positions, the anatomy of the muscle group, the landmarks of good soreness/bad soreness, etc., should refer back to the extensive information in Section 3.

The soleus muscle and the hip flexors (the psoas and the iliacus muscles) are not included in this section. I have reservations about the importance and the positioning of the soleus stretch. I certainly believe that the hip flexor stretch needs to be done carefully, and only after reviewing all the information in Section 3.

Also, it is important for everyone to remember to warm up before stretching.

I. GASTROCNEMIUS STRETCH: BOTH LEGS AT THE SAME TIME

Isolate the Muscle Group

- The best position to isolate the gastrocnemius muscles is standing with the entire ball of both feet resting on a raised surface and the heels firmly weight-bearing on the ground.

Find Zero Tension

- Lean backward, away from the door frame or whatever you are holding onto, to reduce the gastrocnemius muscle tension to zero.

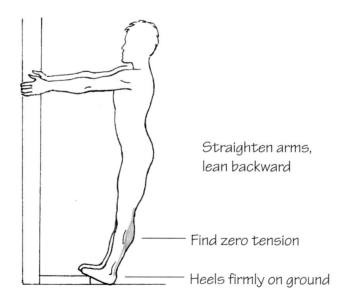

Straighten arms, lean backward

Find zero tension

Heels firmly on ground

Find the First Awareness

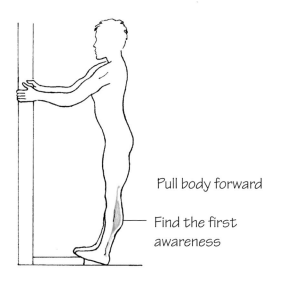

- Once you have reached "zero tension" by leaning backward, slowly pull your body forward with your arms until you feel the first gentle tension in the middle of the gastrocnemius muscles.

Pull body forward

Find the first awareness

Less is Best

- There should be no sensation of pulling or tension behind the knee.
- You will usually feel one gastrocnemius muscle more than the other. The difference you feel is the best biofeedback of these muscles you can have.
- Don't go past that point until the tension is gone.

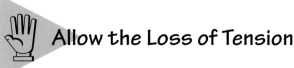

Allow the Loss of Tension

- Hold that position and allow that first tension to diminish and release.
- Repeat the sequence by pulling forward and finding the second gentle tension in the calf muscles.

II. SITTING GROIN STRETCH: (SITTING ADDUCTOR STRETCH)

Isolate the Muscle Group

- To isolate the adductors the stretch should be done sitting.
- Rest the back against a wall and place the heels together, allowing the legs to fall laterally as illustrated.
- If there is nothing to lean your back against, use your arms to support the body, and keep the back straight.

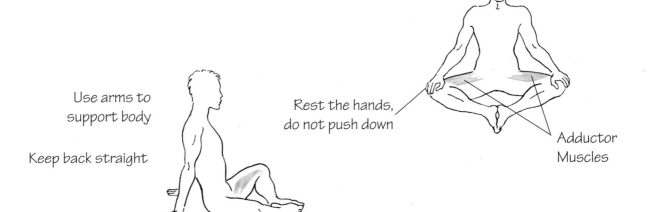

Use arms to support body

Keep back straight

Rest the hands, do not push down

Adductor Muscles

Find Zero Tension

- Start with the feet far enough from the body that there is no awareness of tension in the groin muscles.

Find the First Awareness

■ Bring the feet toward the pelvis a little at a time until that first gentle tension is felt in the groin muscles.

Less is Best

■ You may feel tension only in one leg initially. That leg has the shorter muscle group. Do not change position until the tension is gone.
■ The goal is more length in the shorter muscle group and more symmetry with the opposite leg.

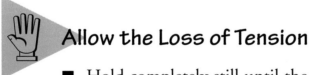

Allow the Loss of Tension

■ Hold completely still until the tension in the groin muscle can no longer be felt.
■ Repeat the stretch a second time.

III. QUADRICEPS STRETCH: LYING ON YOUR SIDE

 ## Isolate the Muscle Group

- The best position to isolate the quadriceps is lying on your side, as illustrated.
- Flex the knee and hold the leg you are stretching just above the ankle; do not hold the foot.

Thigh in Alignment with Body

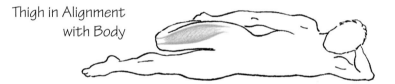

 ## Find Zero Tension

- Start with the thigh far enough in front of the pelvis that there is no awareness of tension in the quadricep muscles.

Find the First Awareness

- Find the first gentle tension in the middle of the quadriceps by pulling the leg back with your hand.

- Only a few people with excellent quadriceps length will need to pull the leg behind the pelvis to find the first awareness.

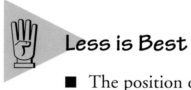

Less is Best

- The position of the leg when you find the first tension does not matter.

Allow the Loss of Tension

- Hold that position until the tension in the quadriceps is gone.

- Repeat this sequence with the other leg.

IV. SITTING HAMSTRING STRETCH

Isolate the Muscle Group

- To isolate the left hamstring muscles, sit in the position illustrated.
- The left leg should be at a 90-degree angle to the pelvis.
- Use the arms to support the upper body with the back straight.

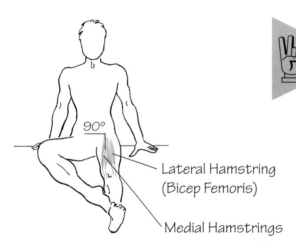

90°

Lateral Hamstring
(Bicep Femoris)

Medial Hamstrings

**Anterior (Frontal) view of hamstring muscles
with femur and all other muscles removed**

Find Zero Tension

- Move the arms and upper body backward until there is no awareness of tension in the hamstrings.

Find the First Awareness

- Move the arms and upper body forward to find the first awareness of tension in the hamstrings.
- Keep the head up and the back straight.

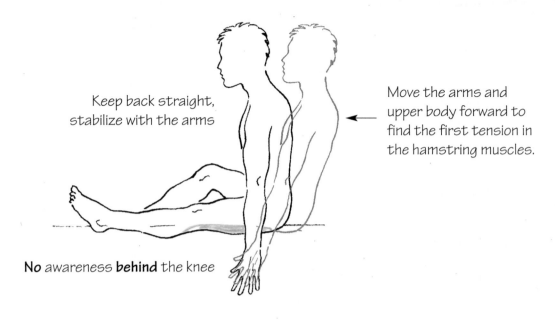

Keep back straight, stabilize with the arms

Move the arms and upper body forward to find the first tension in the hamstring muscles.

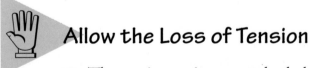

No awareness **behind** the knee

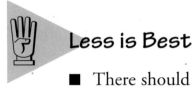

Less is Best

■ There should be no tension behind the knee. The first awareness should be felt in the muscles well above the knee joint.

Allow the Loss of Tension

■ The static tension must be held long enough for the relaxation/sliding elongation to happen.
■ Repeat this sequence with the other leg.

V. GLUTEUS MAXIMUS AND EXTERNAL HIP ROTATOR STRETCH

Isolate the Muscle Group

■ The best position to isolate the gluteus maximus and the external hip rotators of the right hip is lying flat on your back as illustrated

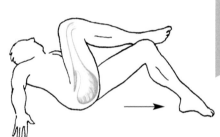

Start where there is no tension in hip muscles

Find Zero Tension

■ If you feel tension in the posterior muscles of the right hip, gradually move the left foot farther from your body until there is no tension.

Find the First Awareness

■ Gradually bring the left foot toward the pelvis until you feel the first awareness of tension in the posterior muscles of the right hip.

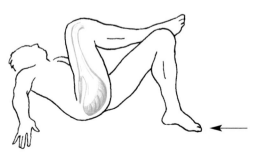

Isolates the gluteus maximus and external hip rotators

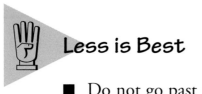

Less is Best

■ Do not go past that position until the first gentle tension is gone.

■ If the first tension has not been found in the posterior muscles of the right hip when the left foot is as close to the body as possible, you must lift the left leg off the ground until you find the first awareness in the right hip muscles.

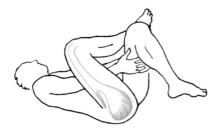

Use hands to life leg by grasping thigh beneath knee

■ Use your hands to lift the leg, grasping the thigh just beneath the knee as illustrated.

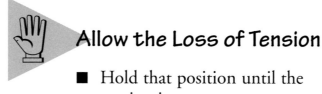

Allow the Loss of Tension

■ Hold that position until the tension is gone.
■ Repeat this sequence with the opposite leg.

NOTES

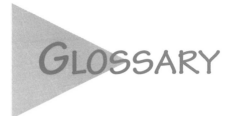

GLOSSARY

Abduction - in biomechanics, a movement away from the midline (center) of the body.

Accelerate - to speed up; quicken.

Actin protein - a protein localized in the I band of the myofilaments contained in the sarcomeres of muscle fibers. Acting along with the myosin protein, it is responsible for the contraction and relaxation of muscle.

Acute - having a short and relatively severe course.

Adduction - in biomechanics, a movement toward the midline of the body.

Anterior - situated in front of or in the forward part of the body; a term used in reference to the ventral or belly surface of the body.

Aponeurosis - a white, flattened or ribbon-like tendinous expansion, serving mainly to connect a muscle with the parts that it moves, e.g., the plantar aponeurosis or plantar fascial.

Articular - a term of or pertaining to a joint, e.g., articular cartilage/joint cartilage.

Articular Cartilage - a thin layer of cartilage, usually hyaline, on the articular surface of bones in synovial joints. This cartilage allows gliding motion in the joints.

Asymmetrical - lack or absence of symmetry; dissimilarity in corresponding parts or organs on opposite sides of the body which are normally alike.

Ballistic movement - a sudden, jerking movement.

Best resting length - when the myofilaments are at their longest possible length in human muscle tissue without stretching.

Biofeedback - a learned response to stimuli; in this book, learning to feel the subtlety and proper location of the tension felt in a muscle or muscle group. This is a conditioned response.

Biomechanics - the application of mechanical laws to living structures, specifically to the locomotor system of the human body.

Body mass - the total weight of the cells of the body.

Calcaneus - the heel bone.

Chondromalacia - premature degeneration of the patellar cartilage caused by chronic inflammation, causing pain when the patella is pressed against or is pulled over the femur.

Chronic - persisting over a long period of time.

Collagen - an albuminoid, a main supportive protein of skin, tendon, bone, cartilage, and connective tissue.

Collagenous fibers - fibers composed of collagen.

Concentric contraction - a shortening contraction of muscle; the muscle is expending energy and producing motion.

Contraction - as applied to muscle function it implies development of tension and the expenditure of energy, regardless of whether the muscle is shortening, elongating, or maintaining constant length.

Current resting length - this refers to the length of the myofilaments of the weight-bearing muscles when they are not expending energy or doing work. The current resting length is seldom the best resting length in these muscles, because they shorten with repetitive usage and fatigue.

Decelerate - to slow down.

Degeneration - deterioration; change from a higher form to a lower form; especially change of tissue to a lower or less functionally active form.

Degenerative - of or pertaining to degeneration.

Dissipate - to reduce and spread, as in spreading the loading force of impact over the largest area of the articular cartilage of the joints.

Dynamic stretches - see page 74, section 2.

Eccentric capacity - this term describes the distance the sarcomeres of a muscle can elongate from their *maximally contracted position* to the point where the overlapping protein fibers slightly exceed their *current resting length* during an eccentric contraction. When the overlapping protein fibers of the myofilaments slightly exceed their current resting length, the muscle spindles cause a myotatic reflex response in the muscle. This stops further elongation of the muscle. This myotatic reflex contraction stops the muscle fibers from overextending and tearing. This reflex contraction in response to loading force and myofilament elongation defines the limits of that muscle's eccentric contraction.

Eccentric contraction - an elongating contraction of muscle; the muscle is expending energy as it elongates to control motion.

Edema - swelling; an accumulation of fluid in the intercellular spaces of the body.

Elastic - susceptible of being stretched, compressed, or distorted, and then tending to assume its original shape; resilient.

Elastic deformity - as pertaining to ligaments, a tear or rupture caused by an acute or sudden overload of the structure that exceeds the structure's tensile strength.

Elastic fibers - fibers composed of the elastin protein.

Elastin - a yellow scleroprotein, the essential constituent of yellow elastic connective tissue; it is brittle when dry, but when moist is flexible and elastic.

Exostosis - a benign bony growth projecting outward from the surface of a bone, usually caused by repetitive external pressure on the bone.

Eversion - in biomechanics, a turning outward, especially of the calcaneus or foot.

Extension - a movement which brings the bones of a limb into or toward a straight condition, e.g., extending or straightening the knee.

External - situated or occurring on the outside; many anatomical structures formerly called external are now more correctly termed lateral.

Fascia - a sheet or band of fibrous connective tissue that forms an investment for muscles and various organs of the body. Muscle fascia surrounds and contains the muscles.

Fasciculi - the large bundles of muscle fibers (myofibrils) encapsulated by individual fascial components (perimysium).

Femur - the bone that extends from the pelvis to the knee, being the longest and largest bone in the body; also called the thigh bone and femoral bone.

Fibrosis - the formation of fibrous tissue; scar tissue.

Fibula - the outer and smaller of the two bones of the lower leg below the knee. It articulates with the lateral aspect of the tibia above and the talus below (forming the lateral aspect of the ankle joint).

Flexion - the act of bending or condition of being bent, e.g., bending or flexing the knee.

Fracture - a break or rupture in a bone.

Hernia - the protrusion of a loop or knuckle of an organ or tissue through an abnormal opening.

Herniated disk - herniation of the intervertebral disk of the spine; the protrusion of the nucleus pulposus or annulus fibrosus of the disk, which may impinge on spinal nerve roots.

Hypermobility - excessive movement in a joint.

Hypertrophy - the enlargement or overgrowth of a bone due to an increase in size of its constituent cells. Bones hypertrophy in response to excess or external stress. This bone growth results in exostosis (i.e. a bunion).

Incontinence - inability to control bowel and/or bladder functions. This can be manifested in many forms.

Inelastic - not elastic; tends not to assume its original shape if stretched or distorted; not resilient.

Inflammation - a localized protective response caused by injury or destruction of tissues. It is characterized in the acute form by pain, heat, redness, swelling, and loss of function.

Inguinal - pertaining to the groin (the inguen).

Inguinal ligament - a fibrous band of connective tissue (a ligament) running from the anterior superior spine of the ileum to the spine of the pubis. This is the largest ligament on the front of the pelvis.

Insidious - coming on in a stealthy manner; of gradual and subtle development.

Internal - situated or occurring within or on the inside; many anatomical structures formerly called internal are now correctly termed medial.

Inversion - in biomechanics, an inward movement, especially of the calcaneus and foot.

Isometric contraction - a static or holding contraction of muscle. The muscle is expending energy and maintaining a position, but the myofilaments are not changing length.

Joint capsule - articular capsule; the sac-like envelope which encloses the cavity of a synovial joint by attaching to the circumference of the articular end of each involved bone; it consists of a fibrous membrane and a synovial membrane. This capsule completely surrounds the joint itself, and functions to support the joint (the fibrous membrane), and to nourish and lubricate the joint (the synovial membrane).

Lateral - denoting a position farther from the median plane or midline of the body or of a structure; pertaining to a side.

Ligament - a band of fibrous tissue that connects bones, serving to support and strengthen joints.

Load - as used in the context of muscle stretching, e.g., loading a muscle, this term identifies the first stress placed on a muscle which results in the reflex contraction of that muscle.

Lower extremity - the leg from the hips down, including the joints of the hip, knee, ankle, and foot.

Lumbar spine - the low back, consisting of the five lumbar vertebrae between the thoracic vertebrae and the sacrum.

Macroscopic trauma - damage or injury to tissue visible with the unaided eye or without the microscope.

Malalignment - displacement out of line, especially of joint position and posture.

Medial - pertaining to the middle; closer to the midline of the body or structure.

Microscopic trauma - damage or injury to tissue visible only by the aid of the microscope.

Momentum - the quantity of motion; the product of mass times velocity.

Muscles - organs which by contraction produce the movements of an animal organism; the contractile tissue of the body.

Myofibril - a muscle fibril, one of the slender threads which run parallel with the long axis of the fiber, and are composed of sarcomeres. Each sarcomere contains two myofilaments.

Myofilament - any of the ultramicroscopic threadlike structures occurring in bundles in the myofibrils of striated muscle fibers. The thick filaments are composed of myosin, the thin ones of actin; together they are responsible for the contractile properties of muscle. Two myofilaments form a sarcomere.

Myosin protein - the most abundant protein (68 per cent) in muscle, occurring chiefly in the A band of the myofilaments of the sarcomere. Acting along with actin protein, it is responsible for the contraction and relaxation of muscle.

Myotactic - pertaining to the proprioceptive senses of muscles; a contraction caused by the proprioceptors of the body in response to gravity, balance, and/or position, e.g., the myotactic reflex response of the hamstrings when bending forward from the waist. The muscle's proprioceptors, aided by other sensory organs in the body, react to gravity and balance by keeping the hamstring contracted to stabilize this posture.

Myotatic - induced by stretching or extending a muscle under load; a contraction caused or induced by stretching or extending a muscle under load, e.g., the myotatic reflex contraction of the gastrocnemius muscle when the overlapping protein fibers of the myofilaments are extended slightly past their current resting length in an eccentric contraction during the gait cycle. Also, it is the first tension (contraction) felt when a muscle is initially loaded during a stretch.

Neuron - any of the conducting cells of the nervous system.

Osgood-Schlatter disease - osteochondrosis of the tuberosity of the tibia; also called apophysitis tibialis adolescentium. This roughly translates to the fact that the patella ligament (quadriceps tendon) causes excess traction on the periosteum of the apophyseal growth plate of the anterior tibia.

Patella - a triangular sesamoid bone situated at the front of the knee in the tendon of insertion of the quadriceps muscles; the knee cap.

Patella-femoral syndrome - inflammation, pain, and degeneration of the articular surfaces of the patella and the femur (the knee cap and knee joint).

Pelvis - the lower portion of the trunk of the body, bounded anteriorly and later- ally by the two hip bones and posteriorly by the sacrum and the coccyx (tail bone).

Periosteum - a specialized connective tissue covering all bones of the body, and possessing bone-forming potentialities.

Plastic deformity - as pertaining to ligaments, a continuous and prolonged stress that causes microscopic tearing, scarring, weakening, and permanent abnormal lengthening of the ligaments. This results in a loss of stability of the joint the ligaments stabilize, resulting in hyper-mobility of the joint.

Pliant - flexible.

Plantar fascia - bands of tendinous tissue radiating toward the bases of the toes from the medial process of the tuber calcanei (the plantar aspect of the heel bone); also called the plantar aponeurosis.

Plantar fasciitis - inflammation of the plantar fascia due to *overload* and *traction* that results in damage to the plantar fascia and to the periosteum of the calcaneus that it arises from.

Posterior - situated in back of, or in the back part of, or affecting the back part of a structure.

Posterior compartment syndrome - damage to the deep posterior compartment of the lower leg. This compartment contains the flexor digitorum longus, flexor hallucis longus, and tibialis posterior muscles, as well as major blood vessels and nerves. Inflammation increases the pressure in this closed space, and can cause severe nerve damage.

Pronation - as applied to the foot, a combination of eversion of the calcaneus and the tarsal joints and abduction of the metatarsal joints resulting in the lowering of the medial longitudinal arch. This happens in the first part of the midstance phase of gait.

Proprioceptive - receiving nerve stimuli within the tissues of the body, as within muscles and tendons.

Proprioceptive Neuromuscular Facilitation (PNF) Stretching - see page 75, section 2.

Proprioceptor - sensory nerve terminals which give information concerning movements and position of the body; they occur chiefly in the muscles, tendons, and the labyrinth of the brain.

Propulsive phase of gait - a term used for the 4th phase of the normal gait cycle, starting when the heel is lifted off the ground, and ending when the ball of the foot leaves the ground.

Resting length of a myofilament - the position of the actin and myosin proteins in the myofilaments when the muscle is not working or expending energy.

Sacrum - the triangular bone just below the lumbar vertebrae (the lower back), formed usually by five fused vertebrae (sacral vertebrae) that are wedged dorsally between the two hip bones.

Sarcomere - the unit of length of a myofibril, being the distance between two Z bands. Two myofilaments are contained in a sarcomere.

Sciatica - a syndrome characterized by pain radiating from the lower back into the buttock and into the lower extremity (the back of the thigh) along its posterior or lateral aspect, and commonly caused by prolapse of the intervertebral disk (herniated disk); the term is also used to refer to pain anywhere along the course of the sciatic nerve.

Sciatic nerve - the largest diameter nerve in the body; it is formed by nerve roots exiting the lower spine at intervertebral levels L4, L5, S1, S2, and S3. This large nerve travels through the posterior aspect of the pelvis and down the back of the thigh. It has many branches throughout these areas.

Sesamoid - denoting a small nodular bone embedded in a tendon or joint capsule; a sesamoid bone.

Sliding elongation of muscle myofilaments - see pages 28-30, section 1.

Static - acting with mere weight without motion; not moving, not active; i.e. static stretches.

Static stretching - see page 78, section 2.

Supination - as applied to the foot, a combination of inversion of the calcaneus and the tarsal joints and adduction of the metatarsals resulting in the raising of the medial longitudinal arch. This should be the second part of the midstance phase of gait.

Swelling - edema of the tissues.

Systemic - pertaining to or affecting the body as a whole.

Tendinitis (tendonitis) - inflammation of tendons and of tendon-muscle attachments.

Tendon - a fibrous cord of connective tissue in which the fibers of a muscle end and by which the muscle is attached to a bone or other structure. A tendon can only elongate 3% of the normal fiber length without rupturing.

Tendon (synovial) sheath - the sheath that surrounds tendons anywhere they are put under traction as they are pulled across a bony prominence. The sheath secretes synovial fluid, which serves as a lubricant as well as nourishes the tendon.

Tenosynovitis (tendosynovitis) - inflammation of a tendon sheath.

Tensile strength - relating to the strength of a tissue when tension is applied.

Tibia - the shin bone; the inner and larger bone of the leg below the knee; it articulates with the femur and head of the fibula above and with the talus below (forming the medial part of the ankle joint).

Velocity - rate of speed.

Vertebra - any of the thirty-three bones of the spinal column, comprising the seven cervical (neck), twelve thoracic (upper back), five lumbar (lower back), five sacral (posterior aspect of pelvis), and four coccygeal (tail bone) vertebrae.

Vertebrae - plural of vertebra.

Vertebral column - the spinal column; the spine.

Viscosity - a physical property of a substance that is dependent on the friction of its component molecules as they slide by one another. In general, viscosity of body tissues drops as the temperature increases, resulting in better function of those structures.

BIBLIOGRAPHY

Alter, Michael J. (1988). *Science of Stretching*. (Champaign, IL: Human Kinetics Publishers, Inc.)

Anderson, B. (1980). *Stretching*. (Bolinas, CA: Sheldon Publications).

Assussen, E. (1956). Observation on experimental muscle soreness. *Acta Rheumatology Scandinavica*, 2, 109-116.

Asmussen, E. & Bonde-Petersen, F. (1974). Storage of elastic energy in skeletal muscles in man. *Acta Physiologica Scandinavica*, 91(3), 385-392.

Basmajian, J.V. (1975). Motor learning and control. *Archives of Physical Medicine and Rehabilitation*, 58(1), 38-41.

Basmajian J.V. (1978). *Muscles Alive*, 4th ed. (Baltimore: Williams & Wilkins Co.)

Beaulieu, J.E. (1981). Developing a stretching program. *The Physician and Sportsmedicine*, 9(11), 59-69.

Boscoe, C., Tarkka, I., & Komi, P.V. (1982). Effects of elastic energy and myo-electrical potentiation of triceps surae during stretch-shortening cycle exercise. *International Journal of Sports Medicine*, 3(3), 137-140.

Bryant, S. (1984). Flexibility and stretching. *The Physician and Sportsmedicine*, 12(2), 171.

Burkett, L.M. (1970). "Causative Factors in Hamstring Injuries", *Medicine and Science in Sports*, Vol. 2, Spring 1970.

Burry, Hugh C. (1969). *"Late Effects of Neglected Soft Tissue Injury"*, Proceedings of the Royal Society of Medicine, Vol. LXII, September 1969.

Cavagna, G.A., Dusman, B., & Margaria, R. (1968). Positive work done by a previously stretched muscle. *Journal of Applied Physiology*, 24(1), 21-32.

Cavagna, G.A., Saibene, F.P., & Margaria, R. (1965). Effect of negative work on the amount of positive work performed by an isolated muscle. *Journal of Applied Physiology*, 20(1), 157-160.

Cerney, J.V. (1963). *Athletic Injuries* (Springfield, IL, Charles C. Thomas).

Ciullo, J.V., & Zarins, B. (1983). Biomechanics of the musculotendinous unit. In B. Zarins (Ed.), *Clinics in sports medicine* (Vol. 2, pp. 71-85). Philadelphia: W.B. Saunders.

Cornelius, W.L. (1983). Stretch evoked emg activity by isometric contraction and submaximal concentric contraction. *Athletic Training*, 18(2), 106-109.

Coville, C.A. (1979). Relaxation in physical education curricula. *The Physical Educator*, 36(4), 176-181.

de Vries, H.A. (1961a). Prevention of muscular distress after exercise. *Research Quarterly*, 32(2), 177-185.

de Vries, H.A. (1961b). Electromyographic observation of the effect of static stretching upon muscular distress. *Research Quarterly*, 32(4), 468-479.

de Vries, H.A. (1962). Evaluation of static stretching procedures for improvement of flexibility. *Research Quarterly*, 33(2), 222-229.

de Vries, H.A. (1966). Quantitative electromyographic investigation of the spasm theory of muscle pain. *The American Journal of Physical Medicine*, 45(3), 119-134.

Eldred, E., Hutton, R.S., & Smith, J.L. (1976). Nature of the persisting changes in afferent discharge from muscle following its contraction. *Progressive Brain Research*, 44, 157-171.

Friden, J. (1984). Changes in human skeletal muscle induced by long-term eccentric exercise. *Cell Tissue Research*, 236(2), 365-374.

Greenlaw, Robert K. (1973). *"Function of Muscles About the Hip During Normal Level Walking — An Electromyographic and Biomechanical Study."* Ph.D. thesis, Queen's University, Kingston, Canada.

Gowitzke, B.A., & Milner, M. (1980). *Understanding the scientific basis of human movement* (2nd ed.). (Baltimore: Williams & Wilkins Co.).

Grant's Atlas of Anatomy (1972). Diagram 213. (Baltimore: Williams & Wilkins Co.)

Hill, A.V. (1956). *"The Design of Muscles,"* British Medical Bulletin No. 12, p. 165.

Hill, A.V. (1961). The heat produced by a muscle after the last shock of tetanus. *Journal of Physiology* (London), 159, 518-541.

Holt, L.E. *Scientific Stretching for Sport (3-s).* Nova Scotia: Sport Research Limited.

Holt, L.E., Travis, T.M., & Okita, T. (1970). Comparative study of three stretching techniques. *Perceptual and Motor Skills,* 21(2), 611-617.

Hough, T. (1902). Ergographic studies in muscular soreness. *The American Journal of Physiology,* 7(1), 76-92.

Janse, J. (1976). *Principles and Practice of Chiropractic,* ed. Roy M. Hildebrandt (Lombard, IL: National College of Chiropractic).

Jencks, B. (1977). *Your Body: Biofeedback at its Best.* Chicago: Nelson Hall.

Jenkins, R., & Little, R.W. (1974). A constitutive equation for parallel-fibered elastic tissue. The Journal of Biomechanics, 7(5), 397-402.

James, Nicholas (1970). "Injuries to Knee Ligaments", *Journal of the American Medical Association.*

Johns, R.J., & Wright, V. (1962). Relative importance of various tissues in joint stiffness. *Journal of Applied Physiology,* 17(5), 824-828.

Karpovich, P.V., & Sinning, W.E. (1971). *Physiology of Muscular Activity* (7th ed.). (Philadelphia: W. B. Saunders).

Kendall, Henry O., Kendall, Florence P., & Boynton, Dorothy (1952). *Posture and Pain* (Baltimore: Williams & Wilkins Co.)

Klein, A., Thomas, L.C. (1932). "Posture and Physical Fitness", *Body Mechanics and Practice* (New York: The Century Co.).

Laban, M.M. (1962). Collagen tissue: Implications of its response to stress in vitro. *Archives of Physical Medicine and Rehabilitation,* 43(9), 461-465.

Larson, L.A., & Michelman, H. (1973). *International Guide to Fitness and Health.* (New York: Crown Publishers).

Leard, J.S. (1984). Flexibility and conditioning in the young athlete. In L.J. Micheli (Ed.), P*ediatric and adolescent sports medicine* (194-210). (Boston: Little, Brown, and Company).

Lewin, M.D. (1944). *Backache and Sciatic Neuritis* (Philadelphia: Lea & Febiger).

Light, K.E., Nuzik, S., Personius, W., & Barstrom, A. (1984). A low-loading prolonged stretch vs high-low brief stretch in treating knee contractions. *Physical Therapy,* 64(3), 330-333.

Moore, M.A., & Hutton, R.S. (1980). Electromyographic investigation of muscle stretching techniques. *Medicine and Science in Sports and Exercise,* 12(5), 322-329.

Moorehouse, L.E., & Miller, A.T. (1971). *Physiology of Exercise.* (St. Louis: C.V. Mosby).

Retzlaff, E.W. et al. (1974). "The Piriformis Muscle Syndrome", *Journal of the American Osteopathic Association* 73: 799-807.

Sapega, A.A., Quedenfeld, T.C., Moyer, R.A., & Butler, R.A. (1981). Biophysical factors in range-of-motion exercise. *The Physician and Sportsmedicine,* 9(12), 57-65.

Schmidt, R.A., "Effects of Positional Tensioning and Stretch on Reaction Latency and Contraction Speed of Muscles", *Research Quarterly,* Vol. 38, 1967.

Schuster, R.O. (1973). *"Overuse Syndromes: Arch Strains, Heel Pains, Shin Splints",* Annual Sports Medicine Seminar, California School of Podiatric Medicine, April 28-29, 1973.

Sheehan, George (1974). "Structural Troubles", *The Complete Runner* (Mountain View, California: World Publications).

Shy Yan Ng, "The Significance of Psoas Myospasm in the Lordotic Compared to the Kyphotic Sacro-Lumbar Spine," *Journal of the American Chiropractic Association*, Vol. 15, No. 10 (October 1978).

Slocum, D.B., James, S.L., "Biomechanics of Running", *Journal of the American Medical Association*, Vol. 205, No. 11, September 9, 1980.

Smith, J.L., Hutton, R.S., & Eldred, E. (1974). Post contraction changes in sensitivity of muscle afferents to static and dynamic stretch. *Brain Research*, 78, 193-203.

Tanigawa, M.C. (1972). Comparison of the hold-relax procedure and passive mobilization on increasing muscle length. *Physical Therapy*, 52(7), 725-735.

Taunton, J.E. (1982). Pre-game warm-up and flexibility. The New England *Journal of Sports Medicine*, 10(1), 14-18.

Verzar, F. (1963). Aging of collagen. *Scientific American*, 208(4), 104-117.

Volkov, M.V. & Mironova, Z.S. (1966). "Prophylaxis and Basic Principles of the Treatment of Trauma in Sportsmen," *"Proceedings of International Congress of Sports Sciences"* (Tokyo: Japanese Union of Sports Sciences).

Walker, S.M., "The Relation of Stretch and Temperature to Contraction of Skeletal Muscle", *American Journal of Physical Medicine*, 1959-60.

Walther, D.S. (1981). *Applied Kinesiology: Basic Procedures and Muscle Testing.* (Pueblo, CO: Systems D.C.).

Weber, S., Kraus, H. (1949). Passive and Active Stretching of Muscles, *Physiotherapy Review*, Vol. 29.

Zohar, J. (1973). Preventative Conditioning for Maximum Safety and Performance. *Scholastic Coach*, May, 1973.

BIOGRAPHY - DR. STEVEN D. STARK

Dr. Steven D. Stark's professional career is marked by constantly challenging old ideas in the fields of sports medicine and biomechanics. He is the first and only podiatrist in the province of British Columbia to specialize totally in sports medicine and functional control, and was the first podiatrist appointed to the Sports Medicine Council of British Columbia.

Dr. Stark opened the Podiatric Sports Medicine Group in Richmond, BC in 1986. This medical practice specializes in the treatment and prevention of injuries that are the result of biomechanical problems. His success has been based on treating patients by using a better biomechanical approach to bone malalignment and muscle imbalances and less focus on the symptomatic joint or muscle group. The response to Dr. Stark's work and his clinic has been overwhelming, attracting patients from all over Canada and the United States, and from as far away as Scotland, Chile, and Barbados. He has helped both amateur and professional athletes with correct stretching techniques that have not only helped to eliminate training errors but also improved performances and prolonged careers.

Born in New Mexico, raised in Texas, Dr. Stark holds Bachelor of Science and Doctor of Podiatric Medicine degrees. He completed a three-year postgraduate surgical residency at the David Grant USAF Medical Center at Travis Air Force Base in California. He immigrated to Canada in 1980.

Dr. Stark has been involved in sports all his life. He was an amateur and professional boxer for almost ten years. His last professional fight was at The Forum in Los Angeles in 1972. He then devoted his attention to his first love, horses, becoming a professional trainer. He still spends much of his leisure time riding and training horses. He also continues to be an active swimmer, cyclist, and hiker. Dr. Stark is a firm believer that the only way to stay in shape and to continue with the activities that mean so much to him is to exercise and build good symmetrical muscle function, strength, and, most importantly, power, through stretching and flexibility.

ORDER FORM

The Stark Reality of Stretching

ALSO AVAILABLE FROM YOUR LOCAL BOOKSTORE

Canada		United States	
Each copy @	$22.95	_____ Copies @ $18.95	US$_____
Plus GST (7%)	1.60		
Total cost per book:	$24.55		
_____ Copies @ $24.55	CDN$_____	Shipping (1st book)	$ 5.95
Shipping (1st book)	$ 5.95	Add $3.00 for each extra book	$_____
Add $3 for each extra book	$_____		
Total enclosed:	CDN$_____	Total enclosed:	US$_____

Make cheque or money order payable to:

The Stark Reality

Ship to:

Name _____

Address _____

_____

Phone (work) _____ (home) _____

THE STARK REALITY CORP.

Suite 1115 - 11871 Horseshoe Way
Richmond, B.C. Canada V7A 5H5
Telephone: (604) 538-5074 or Fax: (604) 538-5063

Thank you for your order!